Materials Horizons: From Nature to Nanomaterials

Series Editor

Vijay Kumar Thakur, School of Aerospace, Transport and Manufacturing, Cranfield University, Cranfield, UK

Materials are an indispensable part of human civilization since the inception of life on earth. With the passage of time, innumerable new materials have been explored as well as developed and the search for new innovative materials continues briskly. Keeping in mind the immense perspectives of various classes of materials, this series aims at providing a comprehensive collection of works across the breadth of materials research at cutting-edge interface of materials science with physics, chemistry, biology and engineering.

This series covers a galaxy of materials ranging from natural materials to nanomaterials. Some of the topics include but not limited to: biological materials, biomimetic materials, ceramics, composites, coatings, functional materials, glasses, inorganic materials, inorganic-organic hybrids, metals, membranes, magnetic materials, manufacturing of materials, nanomaterials, organic materials and pigments to name a few. The series provides most timely and comprehensive information on advanced synthesis, processing, characterization, manufacturing and applications in a broad range of interdisciplinary fields in science, engineering and technology.

This series accepts both authored and edited works, including textbooks, monographs, reference works, and professional books. The books in this series will provide a deep insight into the state-of-art of Materials Horizons and serve students, academic, government and industrial scientists involved in all aspects of materials research.

More information about this series at https://link.springer.com/bookseries/16122

Mamata Mohapatra · Balamati Choudhury ·
Suddhasatwa Basu
Editors

COVID-19 Pandemic

Research and Development Activities from Modeling to Realization

Springer

Editors
Mamata Mohapatra
Department of Hydrometallurgy
CSIR-Institute of Minerals and Materials Technology
Bhubaneswar, Odisha, India

Balamati Choudhury
Centre for Electromagnetics
CSIR-National Aerospace Laboratories
Bengaluru, Karnataka, India

Suddhasatwa Basu
CSIR-Institute of Minerals and Materials Technology
Bhubaneswar, Odisha, India

ISSN 2524-5384 ISSN 2524-5392 (electronic)
Materials Horizons: From Nature to Nanomaterials
ISBN 978-981-16-4371-2 ISBN 978-981-16-4372-9 (eBook)
https://doi.org/10.1007/978-981-16-4372-9

This Springer imprint is published by the registered company Springer Nature Singapore Pte Ltd.
The registered company address is: 152 Beach Road, #21-01/04 Gateway East, Singapore 189721, Singapore

Preface

The global outbreak of SARS-CoV-2, COVID-19 a novel strain of coronaviruses, emerged from Wuhan city of China in December 2019 and was later announced as global pandemic by the World Health Organization on 11 March 2020. Combating the disease is difficult as no specific therapeutics and vaccines are yet available against the novel coronavirus. Hence, early detection and containment of infected individuals is the best possible approach to reduce the spread of the infection. Here, in the chapter summarised, the major diagnostic tools are used for the detection of COVID-19 along with their advantages and disadvantages. Additionally, the potential therapeutic approaches are also discussed with their current developmental status.

In Chap. 2, the diagnostic approaches, therapeutics and vaccine candidates along with their current developmental stages have been discussed. As there is a huge spike in the number of cases every day, early diagnosis of the disease has become a significant need to stop the spread of the virus. The gold standard RT-PCR and other existing techniques are having sensitivity, but they are not able to detect the infection at an early stage. Hence, the development of innovative rapid testing point-of-care device which can detect the disease at its onset with high sensitivity, specificity and reproducibility is the need of the hour. A few of the drug candidates within the two broad categories of therapeutic approaches have the potential to reduce the load of the disease after they clear the clinical trials parameters. But a specific drug against the SARS-CoV-2 may take several years to develop and manufacture at a commercial scale.

Personal Protective Equipment designated as PPE is considered to be the most important protective equipment designed for safeguarding both public and personal health against infectious microbial agents other toxic materials. The third chapter gives an overview about the importance and use of the Personal Protective Equipment (PPE) as corona virus shielding material. The various contents of the chapter focussed on different types of PPE, its formation and preparation. The importance and values of Personal Protective Equipment (PPE) are also included in the chapter. The details of disposing of contaminated PPE are included along with the discussion about annual procurement (demand) for PPE via UNICEF.

The Indian scenarios as well the world scenario about the availability of PPE are also investigated. Also, the future perspective of the PPE market is also discussed. The polymers which are used in the manufacturing of PPE kits take part in a vital character from the prevention of the disease. The global overview is also presented which focuses on the production rate of PPE along with the materialistic points of the polymers which have been used. Globally, the demand for PPE kits is at a high-inclined position since the corona virus pandemic is widely affected.

The research studies focus on the progress of the wide utilization of the antiviral drugs which have potential efficiency for combating the emerging viruses. Cost-effective, easy to synthesise effective antiviral drugs could lessen the burden of the challenges faced worldwide due to the COVID-19 pandemic. Till date, there are no competent antiviral drugs or vaccines available for treating COVID-19. The optimistic results in all the possible areas are explored counting antiviral drugs that are exists for other viral diseases, are subjected to clinical assessment. Material aspects for detection and monitoring related to various diagnostic measures for COVID-19 with and without the aid of nanoparticles have been discussed in Chap. 6. With the day-to-day surge in the affected number of people, it has become utterly important to detect the virus at an early stage. Detection platforms like genome sequencing has high accuracy for diagnose of COVID-19; still, it was not applicable for rapid diagnosis for clinical large samples because of the longer sequencing time and high requirements. Reverse transcription polymerase chain reaction (rRT-PCR) has been massively employed to detect SARS-CoV-2 in public health and clinical laboratories because it a specific and sensitive diagnostic method for detection the novel coronavirus however it strongly relies on complex apparatus, skilled personnel and a continuous power supply and hours of time. In addition, remote areas do not have equipped rRT-PCR diagnostic services. Thus, the need of the hour is to design easy-to-use, fast and more simplistic detection techniques for COVID-19. Recent developments focussing disinfectant systems for effective inactivation of corona viruses are discussed in Chap. 7. Along with the possible measures, disinfectants for inactivation of plausible exposed and high-risk places along with day-to-day sanitising practices can go a long way can repudiate the virus surge. Though there are variety of disinfectants available for inanimate and animate surfaces their appropriate use and dosage is very essential for maximum efficacy and dodging any related human health hazards. This chapter focuses on the various physical and chemical disinfectants available and employed for inactivation of coronaviruses. The optimum dosage and mode of operation along with their efficacies have been elaborated. This chapter is expected to provide a better understanding of the disinfectant technologies available and their suitable dosage for their appropriate use in the foreseen long fight against coronaviruses.

Chapter 8 is based on the using of artificial neural network (ANN) for epidemical outbreaks. The precise forecast informs precautionary of epidemical diseases control. This objective can only be attained through appropriate models. Not only is the forecasting precision essential but also its methodologies and procedure of model selection. This chapter directed on delivering a summary on the application of ANN for the epidemic forecasts. It also proposed a neural network model (multi-layer perceptron feedforward neural network (MLPFFNN)) for the forecasting of new arrival number of COVID-19 cases. A review on the comparison for the achievements of ANN is provided. Hybrid of ANN with other conventional methods are compared. Executing hybrid ANN with advanced algorithms like data transformation, learning algorithm, weight converging optimization increases learning and generalization of ANN beyond training. The proposed model provides a close prediction within a maximum deviation of 1500 cases at the end of July 2020. Chapter 9 discussed the detailed simulation analysis in this chapter on such prevention practices such as ventilation systems, social distances and respiratory mask simulations. In addition to that some of the antiviral material that can be used for antiviral mask production has also been investigated. This chapter tried to summarise some of the simulation studies carried out to assess the efficacy of ventilation systems and the correct use of masks to minimise COVID-19 infection and also tried to integrate some of the studies already done in antiviral materials that can be used in masks and personal protective equipment.

In light of the results of the scientometric analysis of the research paper, in the area of the coronavirus, there was a significant increase in various aspects, which includes the number of author appearances, number of multi-authored articles, etc. In gist, the information on 9257 number of documents related to the above-mentioned research area was extracted from the Web of Science. The extracted information was then used to perform a detailed scientometric analysis and described in Chap. 10. It was observed that the research in this field of study started as early at 2000, but the research in the said field started receiving much attention post-2000. Since then from 2000 till 2020, research articles published reached a number of 9257. United States Department of Health and Human Services being the highest supporter funding agency in coronavirus research among all other agencies globally.

Bhubaneswar, India — Mamata Mohapatra
Bengaluru, India — Balamati Choudhury
Bhubaneswar, India — Suddhasatwa Basu

Contents

About the Editors

Dr. Mamata Mohapatra is currently working as principal scientist at CSIR-Institute of Minerals and Materials Technology, Bhubaneswar. She received her Ph.D. in Chemistry and has post-doctoral experience from the University of Waterloo, Canada. She joined at Hydro and Electrometallurgy department, CSIR-IMMT in 2006 as Junior Scientist and has been undertaking research independently on interdisciplinary field of research in aqueous processing of ores and secondaries, synthesis and surface modification of transition metal oxide/oxalate and carbonate materials for environment and energy application. She has several contributory well-cited publications in international peer review journals in collaboration with IIT Kanpur, Utkal University (India), KIIT, Murdoch University (Australia), and WATLab (Canada). She has successfully supervised several Ph.D./M.Tech./M.Sc. students.

Dr. Balamati Choudhury is Principal Scientist at Centre for Electromagnetics of CSIR-National Aerospace Laboratories, Bangalore, India. She obtained her M.Tech. degree from National Institute of Science and Technology, India and Ph.D. degree in Microwave Engineering from Biju Patnaik University of Technology (BPUT), India in 2013. Her active areas of research and teaching interests are in the domain of soft computing techniques in electromagnetic design and optimization, computational electromagnetics for aerospace applications, metamaterial design applications, RF and microwaves. She was recipient of ICCCES/Outstanding Young Investigator Award in 2016–2017 for her contributions in Metamaterial Science. She was also the recipient of the CSIR-NAL Young Scientist Award in 2013–2014 for her contribution in the area of Computational Electromagnetics for Aerospace Applications. Dr. Balamati has authored or co-authored over 190 scientific research papers and technical reports, besides three books, five Springer Briefs and three book chapters.

Prof. Suddhasatwa Basu is presently Director, CSIR-Institute of Minerals and Materials Technology, Bhubaneswar and also on lien Professor of Department of Chemical Engineering, Indian Institute of Technology (IIT) Delhi. He completed his Ph.D. in Chemical Engineering from Indian Institute of Science (IISc), Bangalore in 1993 and worked as a postdoctoral fellow and as a visiting faculty at University of Alberta, Canada. His broad research interests are in the area of interfacial and electrochemical engineering and their application in hydrogen energy and fuel cell technology. He is Fellow of National Academy of Science of India, Indian Chemical Society and Institute of Engineers and Fellow of Royal Society of Chemistry, UK. He is on the editorial board of many international journals.

List of Figures

Chapter 4

Chapter 5

Chapter 6

Chapter 7

Chapter 8

Chapter 9

Chapter 10

List of Tables

Chapter 8

Chapter 10

Chapter 1
COVID-19 Crisis

Mamata Mohapatra, Arya Das, and Suddhasatwa Basu

1 Introduction

The COVID-19 pandemic has sent tremors around the world causing colossal loss to human lives, still bestowing an unprecedented encounter to public health, lifestyles and economies of the world which already stands gravely affected. One year after the COVID-19 global pandemic, the worldwide lockdowns leave behind immense impact on millions of citizens, shutting down businesses and industries ceasing all the economic commotion. Though the exact economic damage is hard to assess, early estimates by International Monetary Fund predicted a 3% shrink of global GDP in 2020 restated to 4.5% with the course of shutdown of economies with numbers standing at 3.94 trillion US dollars in lost economic output. Developed economies stand hit the most with GDPs of France, Spain and Italy fell by 21.3, 19.2 and 17.5%, respectively. China's GDP dropped by 36.6% in the first quarter of 2020, while India's GDP contracted by a record 23.9% under the impact. As the health and human toll is still on rise, the economic impairment is clearly apparent and embodies the largest economic shudder the world has experienced in decades. Let alone the economic impact the pandemic has left both short- and long-term insinuations for mental health and lifestyles with thousand being unemployed and restricted to their homes.

The mental health impact of catastrophes can outlast the physical impact, several studies point towards the need, and urgency of elevated mental health need will continue well beyond the COVID-19 pandemic itself. The daunting social wreck caused by the pandemic is equally devastating: With predictions of tens of millions

M. Mohapatra (✉) · S. Basu
CSIR-Institute of Minerals and Materials Technology, Bhubaneswar, Odisha 751013, India
e-mail: mamata@immt.res.in

A. Das
Academy of Scientific and Innovative Research (AcSIR), Ghaziabad, Uttar Pradesh 201002, India

M. Mohapatra et al. (eds.), *COVID-19 Pandemic*, Materials Horizons: From Nature to Nanomaterials, https://doi.org/10.1007/978-981-16-4372-9_1

of people are at risk of dwindling into extreme poverty, up to 132 million being undernourished under the influence, which in turn possess a severe risk of increased mortality due to "deaths of despair". The economic depression and social seclusion loom greater danger of drug and alcohol misuse with studies predicting greater fatalities due to suicides. The COVID-19 pandemic stands still as a major health and humanitarian crisis with profound impact on life, health and economy.

The COVID-19 pandemic has sternly injured the world economy with its serious penalties gravely impacting all the countries, societies and individuals all across the globe. Spreading hastily all across borders, the global health catastrophe has turned into a global economic shockwave with stern impact to the vulnerable. Severely paralysing the arteries of global economy, the sustainable economic growth of different economies needs combined global effort with tactful pandemic handling to achieve them. The COVID-19 pandemic has caused significant disruption to developing countries, in particular India, likely to see downward trajectory in economic growth. With production and consumptions scaled back, India sees a greater challenge to revive its already sluggish economy since the implementation of goods and services tax (GST).

The major boom sectors serving as backbone of any economy came to a standstill reporting loss in several thousand crores. The tourism sector has projected an overall loss of US$ 935 billion and possible laying off of 4 crore people related to the sector. With all the international and domestic flights grounded all across the world, the aviation industry stood at a staggering loss of around $370 billion. The agriculture sector though experienced escalation for vegetables, crops, etc. however faced losses forced to reduce prices owing to supply chain issues leading the output to reach markets with inadequate transport availability and labour. The manufacturing units have also suffered substantially in the pandemic with all major consumer electronic firms and automobile firms had to shut down hampering production of essential key products leading to extensive revenue loss. The COVID-19 has also enforced new start-up units to close due to fund unavailability and lack of communication with clients. The shutdown of shopping complexes and theatres and diminishing footfalls even after slow reopening have grossly affected the retail sector with loss and closure putting job of employees at an enormous risk (Fig. 1).

With vaccinations arriving with slow lifting of restrictions, countries have gradually start over their economies, and GDP growth will rely on individual countries' strategies to mitigate the virus via effective vaccination programmes, but the longer-term economic upliftment will hinge on resumptions of jobs and catering unemployment issues across various sectors. With phased vaccination programmes taking place across the world, the rise in cases and the possibility of the second wave hovering do not chalk out stressful conditions deployed as precautionary measure to mitigate the spread and avoid another possible outbreak. For the current emerging market and developing economies, with daunting vulnerabilities in the basket of uncertain future, it is critical to reinforce public health classifications and strong adherence steps against the spread along implementing reforms for stout and sustainable evolution once the health catastrophe subsides. In the race to alleviate

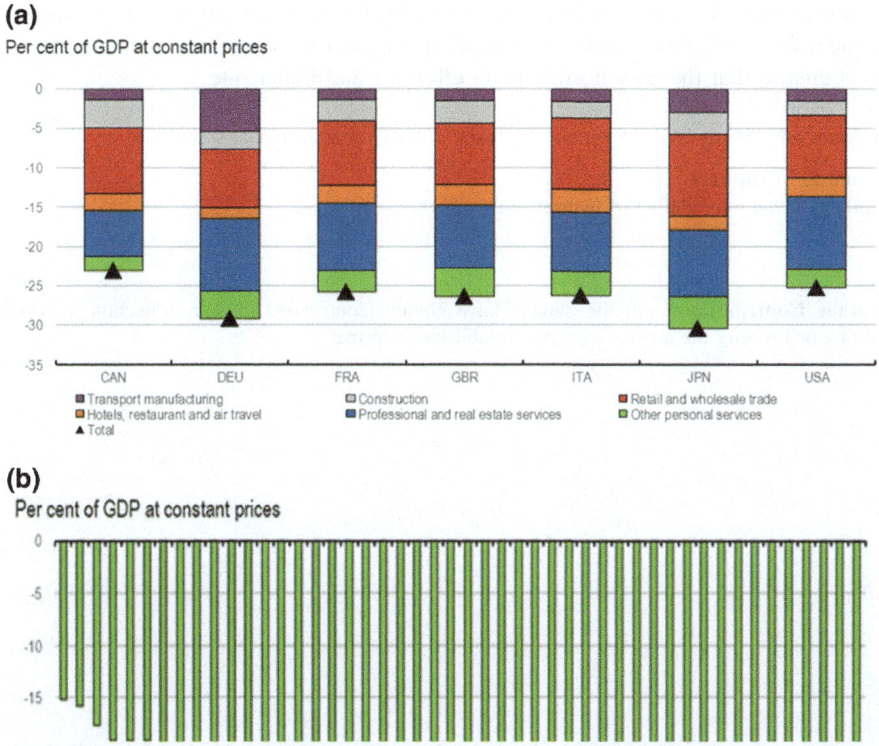

Fig. 1 **a** Initial impact of partial and complete shutdowns on activity major economies and **b** overall loss of major economies. *Source* OECD annual national accounts and OECD calculations, OECD 2020, http://www.oecd.org/coronavirus/en

the loads of the COVID-19 pandemic, it will be pretty vital to consider the augmented necessity for mental health services and to support pertaining the long-term loss and human impact even if the fatality and new infections dwindle. Over the longer prospect, the deep downturns prompted by the pandemic are anticipated to leave behind deep scars through significant attrition of human capital through lost labour, schooling and disintegration of global trade and supply connections all across the globe.

2 Conclusion

The main objective of this chapter is to highlight the need of the hour without overlooking the possibility of another outbreak. The overwhelming situation demands the governments to make noteworthy interventions in response to the current alarming situation and unpredictable future in line with the slow revival of businesses rapidly fine-tuning to the changing needs of the market and customers while traversing to the possible financial, operational and functional challenges to at least ensure that the new normal is an effective and better one.

Acknowledgements All the authors are thankful for their institutional support.

Conflicts of Interest
Authors declare no conflict of interest in this work.

Author Contributions All the authors have equally contributed in data collection, drafting, editing or revising the articles to make it publishable format.

Chapter 2
Deciphering the Recent Advancements in Diagnostic, Therapeutic and Vaccine Candidates Against COVID-19

Arpan Ghosh, Aryan Jaiswal, Nirmal Mohakud, Santosh Kumar Panda, and Namrata Misra

1 Introduction

In December 2019, an outbreak of pneumonia emerged in Wuhan, Hubei Province, China. The rapid rise in acute respiratory failure-related cases in China induced the identification of the causative pathogen as severe acute respiratory syndrome coronavirus 2 or SARS-CoV-2 which have the common clinical manifestations like fever, dry cough and tiredness [1, 2]. WHO declared the outbreak as a global pandemic on March 11, 2020. At present, there are over 190 million confirmed cases globally. Out of these, over 170 million cases recovered and 4 million deceased, with USA leading with almost 35 million cases, followed by India with over 31 million cases and Brazil with over 19 million cases. The novel coronavirus belongs to the *Coronaviridea* family of coronaviruses [3]. Currently, there are seven coronaviruses which commonly infect humans, including 229E (alpha coronavirus), NL63 (alpha coronavirus), OC43 (beta coronavirus), HKU1 (beta coronavirus), MERS-CoV (Middle East respiratory syndrome, beta coronavirus),

A. Ghosh · A. Jaiswal · N. Misra (✉)
KIIT-Technology Business Incubator (KIIT-TBI), Kalinga Institute of Industrial Technology, deemed to be University, Bhubaneswar, Odisha 751024, India
e-mail: namrata@kiitincubator.in

A. Ghosh · A. Jaiswal · N. Misra
School of Biotechnology, Kalinga Institute of Industrial Technology, deemed to be University, Bhubaneswar 751024, India

N. Mohakud · S. K. Panda
Kalinga Institute of Medical Sciences, KIIT deemed to be University, Bhubaneswar 751024, India

M. Mohapatra et al. (eds.), *COVID-19 Pandemic*, Materials Horizons: From Nature to Nanomaterials, https://doi.org/10.1007/978-981-16-4372-9_2

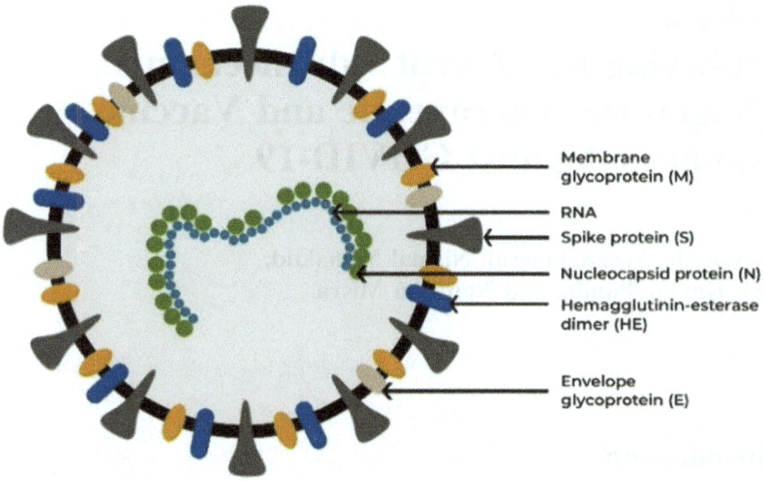

Fig. 1 Schematic diagram of coronavirus structure with surface glycoproteins

SARS-CoV (severe acute respiratory syndrome, beta coronavirus) and SARS-CoV-2 [4, 5]. The SARS-CoV-2 is a single-stranded, positive-sense RNA virus with several glycoproteins like spikes (s) which assist the virus to enter into the host cell, envelope (E) and membrane glycoprotein (M) which plays a significant role in virion assembly and binding of virus particles. Apart from these, there is another glycoprotein called nucleocapsid (N) which packages the viral RNA [6] (Fig. 1). The virus has different sets of genes like ORF-1ab gene that translates a protein which plays a major role in cellular signaling, RdRp gene (RNA-dependent RNA polymerase) which is responsible for replicating virus genetic material inside the host cell, N gene which translates into glycoprotein called nucleocapsid, E gene codes for the envelope for the virus, etc. The RNA virus uses the host cell molecular machinery for replication, due to which it is prone to mutations while transmitting from one animal to another. Genome sequencing analysis of the clinically isolated SARS-CoV-2 revealed by Ren et al on January 25, 2020 [7], initiated various studies on understanding the origin of the virus and also helped to design strategies to fight against the virus. The comparison studies between the novel coronavirus genome with SARS and MERS have effectively led to the identification of many potential therapeutic components and strategies. As there is a rapid surge in the number of positive cases globally, a lot of specific efforts across the globe is being pursued in the search of identifying and developing smart and innovative diagnostic approaches, novel drugs, and safe and effective vaccines to stop, spread and treat the disease. Here, in this chapter, we discussed the current diagnostic approaches to detect SARS-CoV-2 along with the various strategies to develop novel therapeutic candidates including vaccines against the SARS-CoV-2.

2 SARS-CoV-2 Detection Approaches

As the number of positive cases is rising exponentially and there are no specific therapeutic approaches currently available, diagnosing the disease at an early stage becomes very important to contain the disease from community spreading. Currently, there are several methods available to diagnose the disease, but a rapid and sensitive detection approach is still unavailable [8]. The current diagnostic tools are based upon nucleic acid detection (real-time polymerase chain reaction), imaging techniques (Computerised tomography), antigen–antibody reaction (Enzyme linked Immunosorbent Assay), next-generation whole-genome sequencing, etc. (Fig. 2). The real-time polymerase chain reaction (RT-PCR) method is considered the gold standard for SARS-CoV-2 detection.

2.1 Nucleic Acid-Based Detection Techniques

Nucleic acid-based detection uses the DNA/RNA which does highly specific base pairing with the homologous sequences and thus identifies a particular species or subspecies of an organism. The nucleic acid detection includes techniques like polymerase chain reaction (PCR), DNA microarrays, high-throughput whole-genome sequencing, etc. These techniques are faster and provide a lot of information, but they are relatively expensive compared to the conventional culture-based techniques and also require expert manpower to perform the tests. Currently, RT-PCR (TaqMan probe-based) is being used widely for the diagnosis of COVID-19 because of its high sensitivity and specificity. As soon as the genetic sequence of SARS-CoV-2 was released, diagnostic RT-PCR assays were designed based upon the sequence and are made available in the market. A different set of genes like

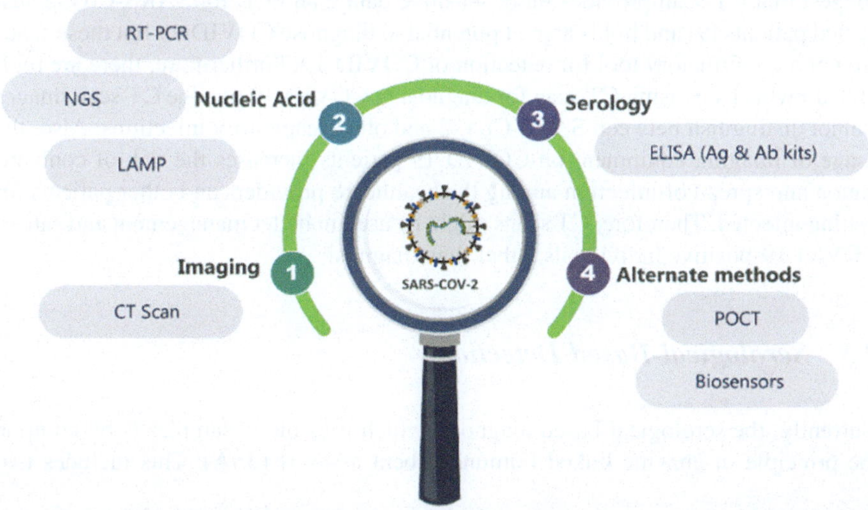

Fig. 2 Schematic representation of COVID-19 diagnosis approaches

ORF-1a gene, ORF-1b gene, RdRp gene, N gene, E gene, etc., are targeted for the detection process. The test generally includes two-step screening, and the target gene for the first step is the highly specific E gene followed by a confirmatory assay with targeted RdRp gene or N gene or ORF-1b. These assays are highly specific and accurate but are very laborious and expensive as well.

One of the promising alternatives to RT-PCR is loop-mediated isothermal amplification (LAMP), but it is still under the process of approval. LAMP is based upon the principle of strand displacement by DNA polymerase at a constant temperature of 60–65 °C eliminating the use of thermocycler. LAMP is a user-friendly technique which can amplify more than 10^9 copies of target sequence at less than an hour time [9, 10]. Also, the combination assay of isothermal amplification and clustered regularly interspaced short palindromic repeats (CRISPR) has emerged as diagnostic tools for the rapid detection of SARS-CoV-2 and requires only lateral flow dipstick for visual detection [11, 12].

Additionally, next-generation sequencing using the nanopore target sequencing plays a great role in the diagnosis of COVID-19. This technique can be used to determine genomic sequences of millions of base pairs in a single experimental setup. Therefore, this technology has great potential to identify unknown organisms including pathogens in a short span of time, but the technology is costly and requires experienced professionals for handling.

2.2 *Imaging Technique—CT Scan*

Early detection of COVID-19 plays a crucial role in the treatment and control of the disease. The nucleic acid techniques are effective when clinical symptoms appear in a patient. But computed tomography (CT) scan usually gives highly sensitive results even before the clinical symptoms appear in COVID-19 patients and can help in early detection of COVID-19 especially in highly pandemic areas [13]. Previous reports suggest that CT scan provides more sensitive data than PCR for SARS-CoV-2 suspected patients [9] and holds a great potential to diagnose COVID-19 but these scans are not a confirmatory tool for detection of COVID-19. Furthermore, there are multiple drawbacks in using CT scan for diagnosing COVID-19 like the CT scan images cannot distinguish between SARS-CoV-2 and other respiratory infections. Also, the usage of imaging equipment on COVID-19 patients increases the risk of contamination and spread of infection among the healthcare providers and other patients for getting infected. Therefore, CT scans might be used in better management and care of COVID-19-positive individuals rather than diagnosis.

2.3 *Serological-Based Detection*

Currently, the serological-based diagnosis which uses blood samples is based upon the principle of enzyme-linked immunosorbent assay (ELISA). This includes two types of tests—detection of antigen (viral components like spike and nucleocapsid proteins) is present in a measurable concentration in the infected patient during the time of infection, and the other one is the detection of antibodies which significantly appears in patients at the later stage in result of immune response against the virus. The two major types of antibodies which are used for detection are immunoglobulin M (IgM) which acts as the first line of defense and appears within a few days of infection and immunoglobulin G (IgG) which plays a major role in the clearance of the infection [14]. There are several antigen and antibody kits developed across the globe like Mylab's PathoCatch, Innovita Rapid Test Kit, etc., but only a few are in the market due to a lack of distribution strategy in the commercialization stage of the devices. These ELISA-based detection kits showed good sensitivity, but they are not useful in early detection of COVID-19 [15, 16].

2.4 Point-of-Care Testing (POCT) Approaches

The handheld POCTs are user-friendly and cost-effective devices that can be used without any expert or professional interventions. These devices generally include various types of biosensors. Biosensors are widely used to detect various infectious diseases like hepatitis, HIV, malaria, etc. At present, these advanced biosensor-based detection approaches are used to build different innovative POCTs which can overcome the limitations of other detection techniques available for diagnosis of COVID-19. One of these innovative devices includes nanomaterial-based biosensors which are highly sensitive because of their high surface-to-volume ratio [17]. The other one in this category includes aptamer-based biosensors which consist of an oligonucleotide having high specificity toward the target molecule (virus particles or antibodies or biomarkers) [18]. Currently, the aptamer-based biosensors are under the developmental phase which can give results within few seconds only.

With the rapid spread of COVID-19 across the globe, the commercial-scale development of alternative methods like rapid antigen–antibody kits, nanomaterials-based biosensors, aptamer-based biosensors, etc., for mass screening with high specificity and sensitivity has become an utter need for the current situation. These technologies can play a significant role in identifying and managing the spread of COVID-19.

3 Therapeutic Approaches Against SARS-CoV-2

Presently, there is no specific drug which can efficiently treat the COVID-19 disease. Many researchers across the globe are working on finding the potential drug components against the SARS-CoV-2. However, such drugs will take several years to develop on a commercial scale. Nonetheless, few existing antiviral drug candidates have shown some therapeutic properties for the treatment of COVID-19.

These antiviral drugs can be broadly divided into two categories based upon their targets. One category includes therapeutic candidates that can directly act on the SARS-CoV-2 and the other that controls the human immune system [19]. Generally, the drugs which target the coronavirus directly interfere with the viral replication mechanism, and on the other hand, the human immune system modulating drugs either boosts the immune response against the virus or inhibits the cytokine storm to prevent lung damage. The major drug candidates against novel coronavirus (nCoV-2) which are under development are discussed.

3.1 Remdesivir

Remdesivir (Fig. 3) is a broad-spectrum pro-drug of an adenosine triphosphate analog and an antiviral agent against RNA viruses which was designed to control the Ebola outbreak. The remdesivir blocks viral replication by inhibiting the RNA-dependent RNA polymerase and is safe for use in humans [20]. According to in vitro studies, remdesivir exhibited inhibitory properties against the SARS-CoV-2 [21]. Currently, remdesivir is under Phase 3 of the clinical trial in multiple countries.

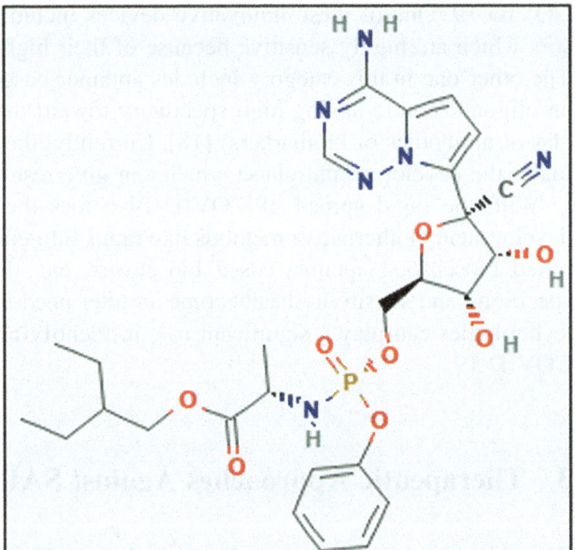

Fig. 3 2-D chemical structure of remdesivir. *Source* NCBI, PubChem [22–27]

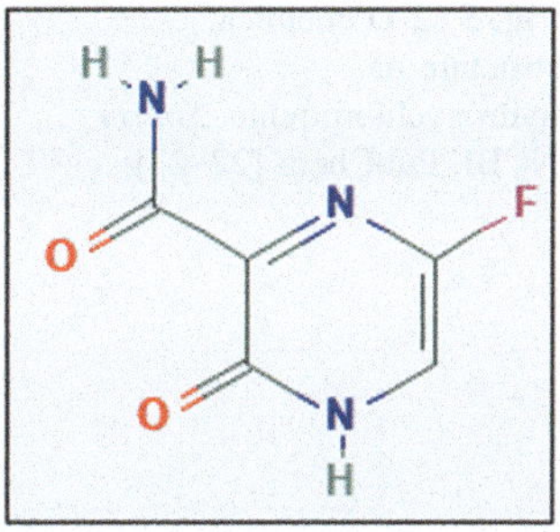

Fig. 4 2-D chemical structure of favipiravir. *Source* NCBI, PubChem [22–27]

3.2 *Favipiravir*

Favipiravir (Fig. 4) is a pyrazinecarboxamide derivative and a broad-spectrum oral RNA-dependent RNA polymerase inhibiting antiviral drug which blocks the viral replication in host cells [28]. Generally, the favipiravir is used to treat influenza infections. Recently, Glenmark Pharmaceuticals got the regulatory clearance to manufacture and market favipiravir under the brand name FabiFlu for the treatment of mild-to-moderate COVID-19 patients.

3.3 *Hydroxychloroquine*

Hydroxychloroquine (Fig. 5) is a 4-aminoquinoline which is widely used as anti-malarial and immunosuppressive agent. It generally makes an alkaline pH in endosomes which inhibits the fusion of membranes between virus and host cell and eventually blocks the entry of the virus [29]. Hydroxychloroquine specifically interferes with angiotensin-converting enzyme-2 (ACE2) [30] which is one of the functional cellular receptors of SARS-CoV-2 [31]. But recently, World Health Organization (WHO) halted the use of hydroxychloroquine for treatment of COVID-19 stating that the drug is not effective against SARS-CoV-2 and fails to reduce the mortality rate of the disease. Food and Drug Administration (FDA) also stated that there have been severe cardiac issues and other side effects of hydroxychloroquine when used for treating COVID-19 patients.

3.4 *Thalidomide*

Thalidomide (Fig. 6) is a glutamic acid derivative which has emerged as one of the potential anti-inflammatory agents which can reduce the formation of TNF-alpha during any inflammatory disease [32]. Additionally, thalidomide also reduces the cytokine level produced in inflammatory response. Currently, thalidomide is under

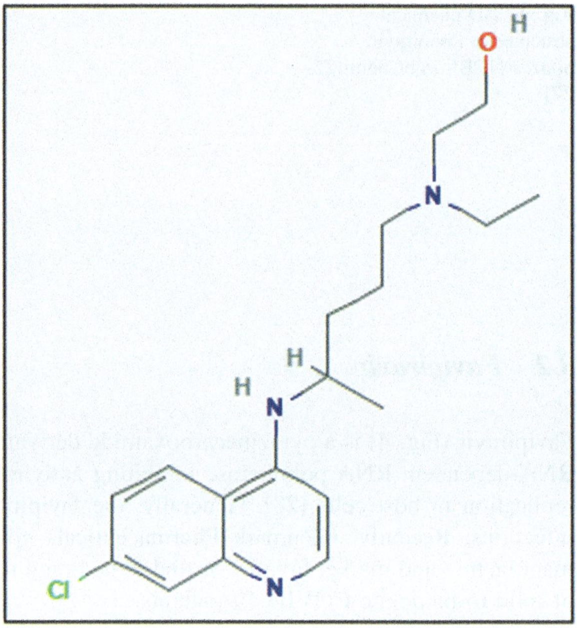

Fig. 5 2-D chemical structure of hydroxychloroquine. *Source* NCBI, PubChem [22–27]

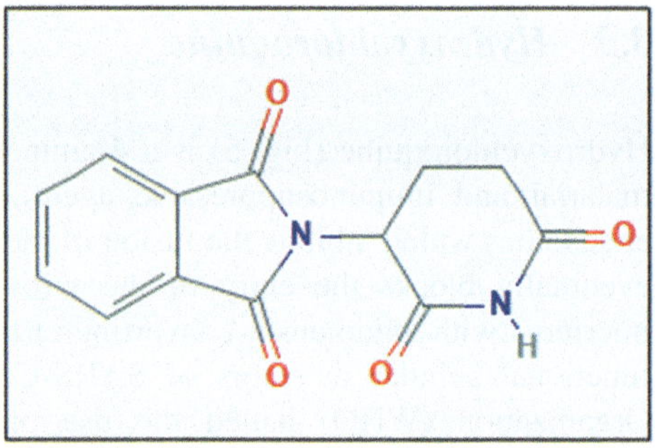

Fig. 6 2-D chemical structure of thalidomide. *Source* NCBI, PubChem [22–27]

clinical studies to check their efficacy in reducing lung damage caused by over-expression of immune response against the SARS-CoV-2.

3.5 *Lopinavir and Ritonavir*

Both lopinavir (Fig. 7) and ritonavir (Fig. 8) are two widely used protease inhibitors which are used in combination for the treatment of HIV infection. Earlier studies have shown that the combinational therapy of lopinavir and ritonavir resulted to be effective against SARS and MERS [21, 28, 33]. However, the clinical trials done on

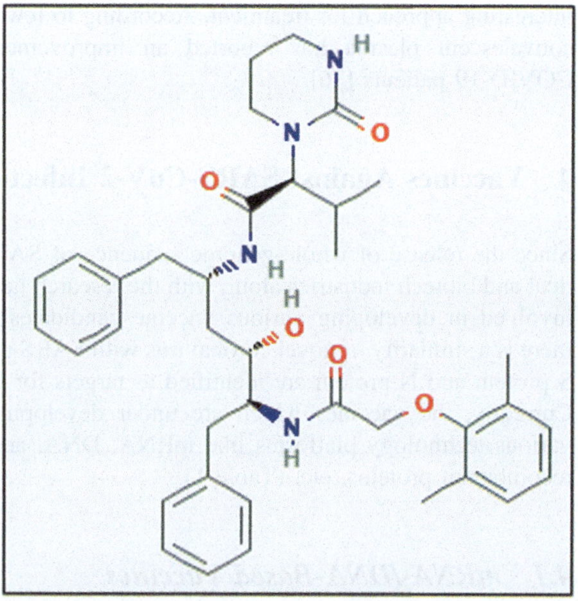

Fig. 7 2-D chemical structure of lopinavir. *Source* NCBI, PubChem [22–27]

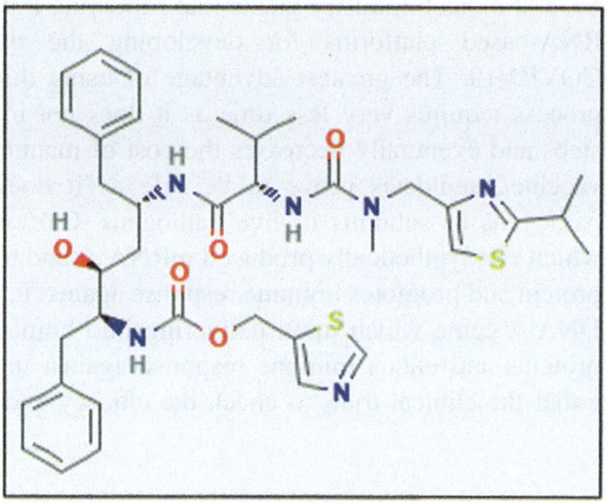

Fig. 8 2-D chemical structure of ritonavir. *Source* NCBI, PubChem [22–27]

mild-to-moderate COVID-19 patients indicated that the combinational therapy of lopinavir and ritonavir is not very effective against SARS-CoV-2 infection [34, 35].

3.6 Convalescent Plasma Therapy

Plasma therapy using the isolated blood plasma from COVID-19-recovered patients which generally contains the neutralizing antibodies against the SARS-CoV-2 is an interesting approach for treatment. According to few studies, the administration of convalescent plasma has reported an improvement in the clinical status of COVID-19 patients [36].

4 Vaccines Against SARS-CoV-2 Infection

Since the release of whole-genome sequence of SARS-CoV-2, many pharmaceutical and biotech industries along with the research laboratories across the globe are involved in developing various vaccine candidates against SARS-CoV-2. Since there is a similarity of novel coronavirus with SARS and MERS at the genetic level, S protein and N protein are identified as targets for COVID-19 vaccines [37, 38]. Currently, the vaccines which are under developmental stages are based upon various technology platforms like mRNA, DNA, adenoviral vectors, subunit and recombinant proteins, etc. (Table 1).

4.1 mRNA-/DNA-Based Vaccines

Several biotech industry giants like Moderna, Inovio, etc., are using the DNA- and RNA-based platforms for developing the potential vaccine candidates for COVID-19. The greatest advantage of using this platform is that the production process requires very less time as it does not involve culturing and fermentation steps and eventually decreases the cost of manufacturing as well [39]. Also, these vaccine candidates prove to be safe as it does not consist of any inactivated pathogens or subunits of live pathogens. Currently, the Moderna's mRNA-1273 which is a synthetically produced mRNA strand translates into stabilized viral spike protein and promotes immune response against it. Similarly, Inovio's INO-4800 is a DNA vaccine which upon delivering into human cells translates into stable viral proteins and elicits immune response against it. Both the vaccine candidates are under the clinical trials to check the efficacy and safety.

4.2 Adenoviral Vectors

Non-replicating adenoviral vectors are one of the powerful vaccination tools against pathogens. The ChAdOx1 nCoV-19 developed by the University of Oxford in partnership with AstraZeneca consists of non-replicating adenovirus, and spike protein sequence of SARS-CoV-2 is under the final stages of clinical trials. The non-replicating adenovirus ensures the safety of this vaccine candidate upon administration in human cells. But the use of adenovirus vaccines can induce immunity against the vector which will eventually reduce the efficacy of the vaccine candidate [40].

Table 1 An overview of major vaccine candidates along with their pros and cons and developmental stage

Vaccine platform technology	Advantages	Disadvantages	Developer and brand name	Developmental status	References
Nucleic acid	• Less time consuming and easy manufacturing • Low manufacturing cost • Ensures maximum safety	• Low efficacy • Multiple dosage requirement	• **Moderna** mRNA-1273 • **Inovio** INO-4800	Clinical trial phase 1	[39]
Adenoviral vectors	• High safety profile • Elicit strong immunogenicity	• May induce immune response against the vector • May induce tumorigenesis	• **University of Oxford and AstraZeneca** ChAdOx1 nCoV-13	Clinical trial phase 3	[40]
Subunit vaccines	• Can be administered in immunocompromised patients • High safety profile	• Low efficacy • May get denatured after administration in human cells	• **University of Queensland**	Clinical trial phase 1	[41, 42]
Live-attenuated virus	• Long-lasting immune response • Low manufacturing cost	• Restricted use in immunocompromised patients • Re-emergence of virulence	• **Codagenix/Serum Institute of India**	Clinical trial phase 3	[43–45]

4.3 Subunit Vaccines

The University of Queensland is currently developing a recombinant viral protein using molecular clamp technology which will remain stable as pre-fusion form of glycoprotein and elicit the production of neutralizing antibodies [41]. But the major challenge with this vaccine candidate is efficacy as it can easily get denatured upon injecting into the human cells [42].

4.4 Live-Attenuated Virus Vaccines

Live-attenuated virus as vaccine candidates is another very promising vaccine development approach and also considered as one of the traditional vaccine development strategies. This platform is based upon the codon deoptimization technology and has shown higher efficacy against respiratory viruses in both in vitro and in vivo experiments [43–45]. This type of vaccine candidates has limited usage in immunocompromised persons and also holds possibilities to get reactivated after administration which puts a big question on its safety profile. Currently, the live-attenuated virus vaccine developed by Codagenix and Serum Institute of India is under the 3rd phase of clinical trials.

5 Conclusion

In this chapter, the diagnostic approaches, therapeutics and vaccine candidates along with their current developmental stages have been discussed. As there is a huge spike in number of cases every day, early diagnosis of the disease has become a significant need to stop the spread of the virus. The gold standard RT-PCR and other existing techniques are having sensitivity, but they are not able to detect the infection at an early stage. Hence, development of innovative rapid testing point-of-care device which can detect the disease at its onset with high sensitivity, specificity and reproducibility is the need of the hour. We can also summarize that a few of the drug candidates within the two broad categories of therapeutic approaches have the potential to reduce the load of the disease after they clear the clinical trial parameters. But a specific drug against the SARS-CoV-2 may take several years to develop and manufacture at a commercial scale. Similarly, we can conclude that many vaccine candidates are in the pipeline of development and regulatory clearance, upon which we can hope that we will get a potential therapeutic resource to halt the current pandemic across the globe.

6 Declaration of competing Interest

The author declares that there is no conflict of interest.

Acknowledgements The author acknowledges the help of Mr. Saikat Gupta, Associate—Design and Campaign, KIIT Technology Business Incubator, Bhubaneswar, in designing one of the pictures in the manuscript.

References

1. Huang C, Wang Y, Li X, Ren L, Zhao J, Hu Y et al (2020) Clinical features of patients infected with 2019 novel coronavirus in Wuhan, China. Lancet 395(10223):497–506
2. Sohrabi C, Alsafi Z, O'Neill N, Khan M, Kerwan A, Al-Jabir A et al (2020) World Health Organization declares global emergency: a review of the 2019 novel coronavirus (COVID-19). Int J Surg
3. Zhang L, Liu Y (2020) Potential interventions for novel coronavirus in China: a systematic review. J Med Virol 92(5):479–490
4. Fehr AR, Perlman S (2015) Coronaviruses: an overview of their replication and pathogenesis. In: Coronaviruses. Humana Press, New York, pp 1–23
5. Basha SH (2020) Corona virus drugs–a brief overview of past, present and future. J Peer Sci 2 (2):e1000013
6. Su S, Wong G, Shi W, Liu J, Lai AC, Zhou J et al (2016) Epidemiology, genetic recombination, and pathogenesis of coronaviruses. Trends Microbiol 24(6):490–502
7. Ren LL, Wang YM, Wu ZQ, Xiang ZC, Guo L, Xu T et al (2020) Identification of a novel coronavirus causing severe pneumonia in human: a descriptive study. Chin Med J
8. Kumar R, Nagpal S, Kaushik S, Mendiratta S (2020) COVID-19 diagnostic approaches: different roads to the same destination. VirusDisease 1–9
9. Notomi T, Okayama H, Masubuchi H, Yonekawa T, Watanabe K, Amino N, Hase T (2000) Loop-mediated isothermal amplification of DNA. Nucleic Acids Res 28(12):e63
10. Dhama K, Karthik K, Chakraborty S, Tiwari R, Kapoor S, Kumar A, Thomas P (2014) Loop-mediated isothermal amplification of DNA (LAMP): a new diagnostic tool lights the world of diagnosis of animal and human pathogens: a review. Pak J Biol Sci 17(2):151–166
11. Esbin MN, Whitney ON, Chong S, Maurer A, Darzacq X, Tjian R (2020) Overcoming the bottleneck to widespread testing: a rapid review of nucleic acid testing approaches for COVID-19 detection. RNA, rna-076232
12. Hou T, Zeng W, Yang M, Chen W, Ren L, Ai J et al (2020) Development and evaluation of a CRISPR-based diagnostic for 2019-novel coronavirus. MedRxiv
13. Chung M, Bernheim A, Mei X, Zhang N, Huang M, Zeng X et al (2020) CT imaging features of 2019 novel coronavirus (2019-nCoV). Radiology 295(1):202–207
14. Long QX, Liu BZ, Deng HJ, Wu GC, Deng K, Chen YK et al (2020) Antibody responses to SARS-CoV-2 in patients with COVID-19. Nat Med 1–4
15. Vogels CB, Brito AF, Wyllie AL, Fauver JR, Ott IM, Kalinich CC et al (2020) Analytical sensitivity and efficiency comparisons of SARS-COV-2 qRT-PCR assays. MedRxiv
16. Okba NM, Muller MA, Li W, Wang C, GeurtsvanKessel CH, Corman VM et al (2020) SARS-CoV-2 specific antibody responses in COVID-19 patients. MedRxiv
17. Liebel M, Hugall JT, van Hulst NF (2017) Ultrasensitive label-free nanosensing and high-speed tracking of single proteins. Nano Lett 17(2):1277–1281
18. Keefe AD, Pai S, Ellington A (2010) Aptamers as therapeutics. Nat Rev Drug Discovery 9 (7):537–550

19. Tu YF, Chien CS, Yarmishyn AA, Lin YY, Luo YH, Lin YT et al (2020) A review of SARS-CoV-2 and the ongoing clinical trials. Int J Mol Sci 21(7):2657
20. Mulangu S, Dodd LE, Davey RT Jr, Tshiani Mbaya O, Proschan M, Mukadi D, Ali R (2019) A randomized, controlled trial of Ebola virus disease therapeutics. N Engl J Med 381 (24):2293–2303
21. Wang M, Cao R, Zhang L, Yang X, Liu J, Xu M et al (2020) Remdesivir and chloroquine effectively inhibit the recently emerged novel coronavirus (2019-nCoV) in vitro. Cell Res 30 (3):269–271
22. National Center for Biotechnology Information (2020) PubChem compound summary for CID 121304016, remdesivir. Retrieved 3 Sept 2020 from https://pubchem.ncbi.nlm.nih.gov/compound/Remdesivir
23. National Center for Biotechnology Information (2020) PubChem compound summary for CID 492405, favipiravir. Retrieved 3 Sept 2020 from https://pubchem.ncbi.nlm.nih.gov/compound/Favipiravir
24. National Center for Biotechnology Information (2020) PubChem compound summary for CID 3652, hydroxychloroquine. Retrieved 3 Sept 2020 from https://pubchem.ncbi.nlm.nih.gov/compound/Hydroxychloroquine
25. National Center for Biotechnology Information (2020) PubChem compound summary for CID 5426, thalidomide. Retrieved 3 Sept 2020 from https://pubchem.ncbi.nlm.nih.gov/compound/Thalidomide
26. National Center for Biotechnology Information (2020) PubChem compound summary for CID 92727, lopinavir. Retrieved 3 Sept 2020 from https://pubchem.ncbi.nlm.nih.gov/compound/Lopinavir
27. National Center for Biotechnology Information (2020) PubChem compound summary for CID 392622, ritonavir. Retrieved 3 Sept 2020 from https://pubchem.ncbi.nlm.nih.gov/compound/Ritonavir
28. Furuta Y, Komeno T, Nakamura T (2017) Favipiravir (T-705), a broad spectrum inhibitor of viral RNA polymerase. Proc Jpn Acad Ser B 93(7):449–463
29. Savarino A, Boelaert JR, Cassone A, Majori G, Cauda R (2003) Effects of chloroquine on viral infections: an old drug against today's diseases. Lancet Infect Dis 3(11):722–727
30. Vincent MJ, Bergeron E, Benjannet S, Erickson BR, Rollin PE, Ksiazek TG et al (2005) Chloroquine is a potent inhibitor of SARS coronavirus infection and spread. Virol J 2(1):1–10
31. Li W, Moore MJ, Vasilieva N, Sui J, Wong SK, Berne MA et al (2003) Angiotensin-converting enzyme 2 is a functional receptor for the SARS coronavirus. Nature 426(6965): 450–454
32. Vargesson N (2015) Thalidomide-induced teratogenesis: history and mechanisms. Birth Defects Res C Embryo Today 105(2):140–156
33. Holshue ML, DeBolt C, Lindquist S, Lofy KH, Wiesman J, Bruce H et al (2020) First case of 2019 novel coronavirus in the United States. New Engl J Med
34. Agostini ML, Andres EL, Sims AC, Graham RL, Sheahan TP, Lu X et al (2018) Coronavirus susceptibility to the antiviral remdesivir (GS-5734) is mediated by the viral polymerase and the proofreading exoribonuclease. MBio 9(2)
35. Cao B, Wang Y, Wen D, Liu W, Wang J, Fan G et al (2020) A trial of lopinavir–ritonavir in adults hospitalized with severe Covid-19. New Engl J Med
36. Shen C, Wang Z, Zhao F, Yang Y, Li J, Yuan J et al (2020) Treatment of 5 critically ill patients with COVID-19 with convalescent plasma. JAMA 323(16):1582–1589
37. Wang N, Shang J, Jiang S, Du L (2020) Subunit vaccines against emerging pathogenic human coronaviruses. Front Microbiol 11:298
38. Jiang S, Du L, Shi Z (2020) An emerging coronavirus causing pneumonia outbreak in Wuhan, China: calling for developing therapeutic and prophylactic strategies. Emerg Microbes Infect 9(1):275–277
39. Le TT, Andreadakis Z, Kumar A, Roman RG, Tollefsen S, Saville M, Mayhew S (2020) The COVID-19 vaccine development landscape. Nat Rev Drug Discov 19(5):305–306

40. Folegatti PM, Ewer KJ, Aley PK, Angus B, Becker S, Belij-Rammerstorfer S et al (2020) Safety and immunogenicity of the ChAdOx1 nCoV-19 vaccine against SARS-CoV-2: a preliminary report of a phase 1/2, single-blind, randomised controlled trial. Lancet
41. Chappell K, Watterson D, Young P (2018) Rapid response pipeline for stabilized subunit vaccines
42. WHO: MODULE 2: Types of Vaccine and Adverese Reactions (2020) https://www.who.int/vaccine_safety/initiative/tech_support/Part-2.pdf
43. Le Nouën C, Collins PL, Buchholz UJ (2019) Attenuation of human respiratory viruses by synonymous genome recoding. Front Immunol 10:1250
44. Mueller S, Stauft CB, Kalkeri R, Koidei F, Kushnir A, Tasker S, Coleman JR (2020) A codon-pair deoptimized live-attenuated vaccine against respiratory syncytial virus is immunogenic and efficacious in non-human primates. Vaccine
45. Nogales A, Baker SF, Ortiz-Riaño E, Dewhurst S, Topham DJ, Martínez-Sobrido L (2014) Influenza A virus attenuation by codon deoptimization of the NS gene for vaccine development. J Virol 88(18):10525–10540

Chapter 3
Personal Protective Equipment (PPE) as Coronavirus Shielding Material

A. K. Srivastava, Sarika Verma, Medha Mili, S. A. R. Hashmi, Rashmi Chowdhary, and Vaishnavi Hada

1 Introduction

Coronavirus (CoVs) is enveloped, non-segmented, positive sense spherical viruses, belonging to the order of *Nidovirales* and family of *Coronaviridae* of about 65–125 nm in diameter. CoVs are the RNA viruses which have the wide genetic data, with genetic data sizes which vary from 26 to 32 kilobases (kb) in length, respectively [1]. The primary target of the coronaviruses includes the respiratory system which, in turn, results in breathing problems in humans. When an infected person coughs, sneezes, or speaks, the droplets which come outside are the main cause behind the spread of COVID-19 [2]. The coronaviruses which are RNA viruses once enter the human cells, first attack the cytokine release which gives signal to T-cell for the proceeding actions (being the central cells for all the viral diseases). Their trimeric spike glycoproteins stick to the cell surface. SARS-CoV-2 ties up with angiotensin-converting enzyme 2 (ACE2) to the human cell surface with elevated connection as compared to other viruses which were responsible for severe acute respiratory syndrome (SARS) in 2003 and middle east respiratory syndrome (MERS). COVID-19 being a global pandemic now and thus is the need of the hour to slow down or prevent its rapid spread until the development or deployment of some effective control measures such as a vaccine. Based on the current evidence, the mode of transmission of this highly contagious deadly SARS-CoV-2 virus from human-to-human is either by direct touch or through

A. K. Srivastava · S. Verma (✉) · M. Mili · S. A. R. Hashmi · V. Hada
Council of Scientific and Industrial Research-Advanced Materials and Processes Research Institute (AMPRI), Hoshangabad Road, Bhopal, M.P 462020, India
e-mail: sarika.verma@ampri.res.in

R. Chowdhary
Department of Biochemistry, All India Institute of Medical Sciences (AIIMS), Bhopal, M.P 462020, India

M. Mohapatra et al. (eds.), *COVID-19 Pandemic*, Materials Horizons: From Nature to Nanomaterials, https://doi.org/10.1007/978-981-16-4372-9_3

contaminated droplets, mainly through respiratory droplets when people cough, sneeze, or exhale infected respiratory droplets [3, 4].

Under these circumstances, PPEs are designated as the most vital equipment which is basically designed for safeguarding both public and personal health against infectious microbial agents. PPE acts as a barrier and is helpful in shielding the infectious coronavirus as well as takes care of the safety of the frontline healthcare personnel like doctors, nurses, other caregivers in this pandemic stage of COVID-19 entries especially in hospital wards, quarantine centres, and primary health centres or testing laboratories [5]. As reported by Food and Drug Administration (FDA), PPE is actually assigned as a strong shielding linking the user's skin, nose, eyes, mouth, or bacterial as well as viral infections or eyes and viral and bacterial infections. They are fabricated specially to protect the health workers from the direct exposure.

Few researchers have reported about PPE in their work like Casanova et al. reported coronavirus survival on healthcare personal protective equipment [6]. Balkhyour et al. reported the evaluation of PPE use and professional subjections in small-scale companies in Jeddah: Health involvement for labourers [7]. Bajwa et al. investigated on peri-operative and critical care concerns in coronavirus pandemic [8]. Rowan et al. studied the challenges and solutions for addressing critical shortage of supply chain for personal and protective equipment (PPE) arising from coronavirus disease (COVID-19) pandemic—case study from the Republic of Ireland [1]. Cook presented on PPE during the COVID-19 pandemic—a narrative review [9].

2 Types of Personal Protective Equipment (PPE)

Personal protective equipment (PPE) are, namely of three types, industrial PPE, healthcare PPE, and consumer PPE as depicted in Fig. 1. The PPE can be respiratory PPE as well as dermal PPE.

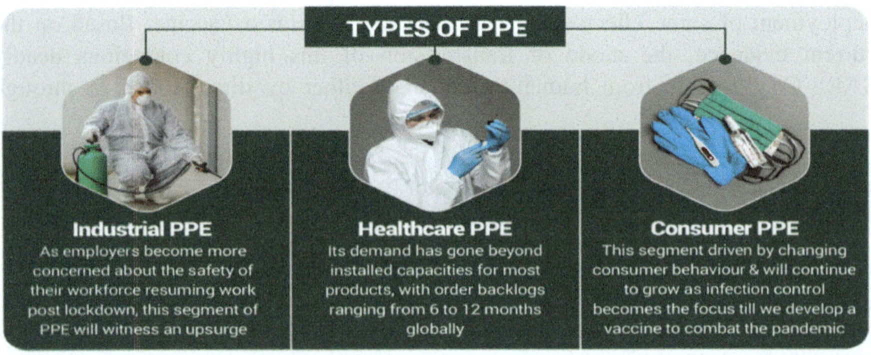

Fig. 1 Various types of PPE available

Further, the use of PPE in every situation will be specific to the means of viral contamination and may differ from the healthcare workers, hospital labourers, and patients. The emergence of this virus pandemic has submerged the worldwide manufacturing of these personal protective equipment's kits as very important censorious outcome in combating COVID-19. The PPE kit majorly consists of respirators (N95 or FFP2 standard or equivalent), masks, face shields, gloves, goggles, gowns, coveralls, boots, or closed-toe work shoes. The PPE should be breathable along with fluid and microbial-resistant characteristics certain medical procedures such as during intubation (the process of inserting a tube through a patient's mouth and into their airway) and nebulizer treatments (a machine that delivers medicated mist to the lungs), necessitate the compulsory requirement of the use of PPE's [6].

Although a number of international organizations like the World Health Organization, the European Centre for Disease Control, Public Health England, the European Society of Intensive Care Medicine, and Society of Critical Care Medicine have produced guidance related to the PPE and which are broadly consistent too. In nutshell, each organization states that mainly the airborne/in-flight safeguard comprises of fit-tested and fit-checked elevated sieve mask; long-sleeved liquid-resistant gown; goggles or visor; and gloves. Progressively, all advices majorly involve the utilization of FFP2 masks or maybe FFP3 masks, respectively.

The PPEs should be simple to wear and easy to remove after being used up, thereby preventing the contamination of the user especially health workers and its surrounding environment. The risk of contamination mainly occurs if the PPE apparel is improperly removed as experienced from earlier SARS epidemic in Canada, which led to infections in the healthcare workers. Every PPE should be deliberately removed, disposed of immediately and appropriately after use. A proper norm or "buddy system" is recommended for the users of PPE during both the processing of donning (i.e., putting on) as well as doffing (i.e., removing) of PPE. The mechanism behind the shielding of coronavirus with the use of PPE is attributed to its difference in the biological structure and chemical compositions [10].

The centres for disease control and prevention (CDC) have issued certain advices and guidelines for the use of personal protective equipment by healthcare personnel to prevent the exposure due to infectious diseases. The lists of PPEs mentioned below prevent the contagious contact of the infectious virus and the healthcare personal [11].

3 Formation of Personal Protective Equipment (PPE)

The polymeric materials are playing most important role in the formation of PPE kits.

Polymers for PPE

Most of the medical PPE and products which are used by the healthcare workers are usually made up of polymeric plastics. The reason to use this polymeric plastic for PPE is mainly its effectiveness. Plastic can be used in many unique ways; hence, it is very much suitable for the respective motive. As plastics are repellent to chemical and gas, these are the perfect material that is used by medical personnel as they have a risk of getting direct contact with blood and infection-causing diseases. It helps as a safety measure and maintains an immediate contact between doctors and patients. Polymeric PPE manifests unexpected low moisture immersion due to its intrinsic configuration. Consequently, fine electrical sheathe effects are achieved above a broad scale of the moisture and climatic situations.

Following are the list of different types of polymers and their chemical structure used for fabricating various types of personal protective equipment (PPE) which are in demand during this global coronavirus outbreak [12–14] (Table 1).

4 Preparation of Personal Protective Equipment (PPE)

The preparation of appropriate personal protective equipment (PPE) is a very important factor which affects its functionality. The detailed overviews for the preparation of important kinds of PPEs which are highly valuable and are in great order during the coronavirus, COVID-19 outbreak are described below. The PPEs are either respiratory or dermal in nature.

4.1 Respiratory PPE

Medical personnel has to be dressed in various kinds of respiratory PPE which includes respirators, dental, and surgical masks.

Face Mask

It is the most important type of PPE used by the frontline workers as well as non-frontline workers in society. The compulsory use of the face masks as PPE by the frontline health workers as well as the general public to combat the spread of COVID-19 is increasing tremendously. Wearing face masks during this epidemic situation has been recommended as a potential tool to tackle coronavirus spread and has been now made compulsory [15]. They can be categorized as with respirators and non-respirators like surgical masks and cloth masks as shown in Fig. 2.

Respirators

Healthcare workers or those at risk of exposure to airborne or fluid hazards should wear the surgical N95 respirators in sterile environments, as they can filter out potential bacteria and viruses, whereas the non-surgical N95s can be used by frontline healthcare workers not involved in surgery but treating the coronavirus-infected patients. However, in the absence of any respirators, it is advised to opt for the next best protection like face masks by the health workers.

Table 1 List of different types of polymers and their chemical structure used for fabricating various types of personal protective equipment (PPE) [12–14]

S. No.	Name of the PPE	Different types of polymers	Chemical structure of polymers
01	Respirators	Polypropylene	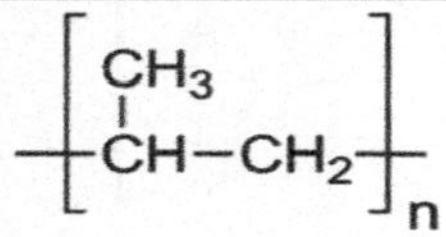 Polypropylene
02	Masks	Non-woven polypropylene and textile material	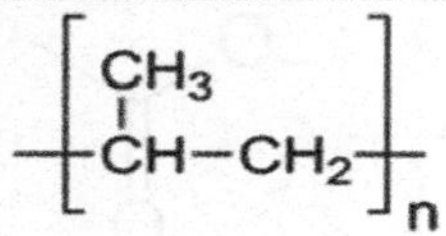 Polypropylene

(continued)

Table 1 (continued)

S. No.	Name of the PPE	Different types of polymers	Chemical structure of polymers
03	Face shields	Polycarbonate, propionate, acetate, polyvinyl chloride, polyethylene terephthalate	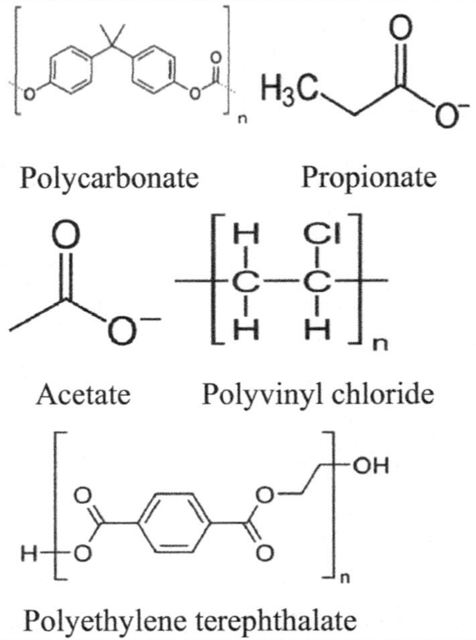
04	Goggles	High purity polycarbonate, neoprene	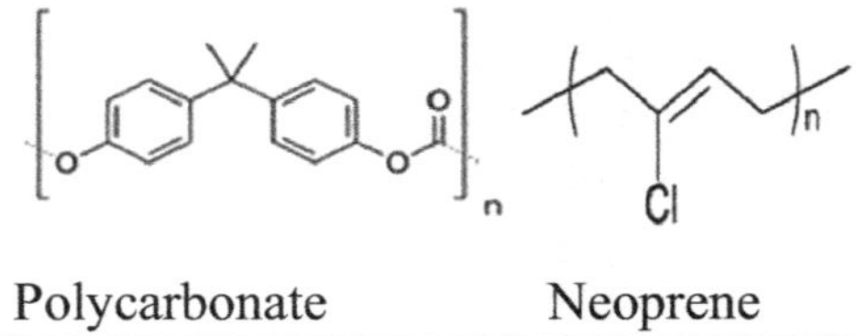

(continued)

Table 1 (continued)

S. No.	Name of the PPE	Different types of polymers	Chemical structure of polymers
05	Gowns	Polypropylene, polyester, polyethylene glycol	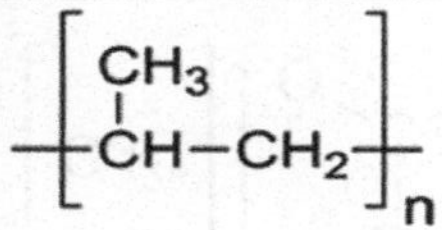 Polypropylene 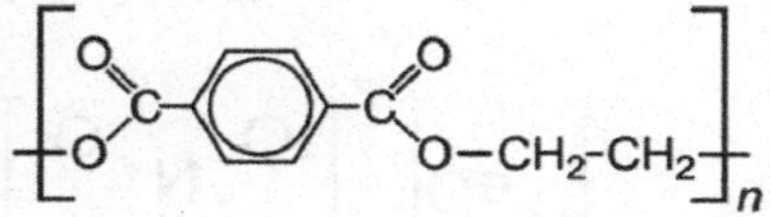 Polyester 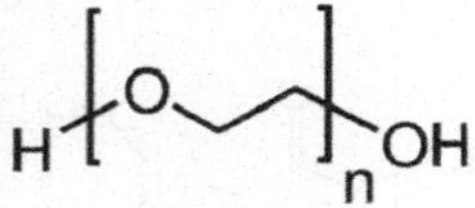 Polyethylene Glycol
06	Coveralls	High density polyethylene	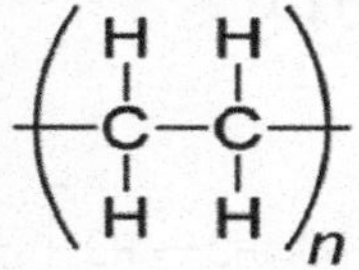 Polyethylene

(continued)

Table 1 (continued)

S. No.	Name of the PPE	Different types of polymers	Chemical structure of polymers
07	Gloves	Rubber, latex, nitrile, calcium nitrate, calcium carbonate	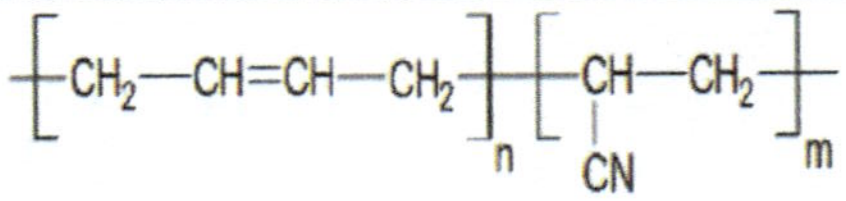 Nitrile Rubber 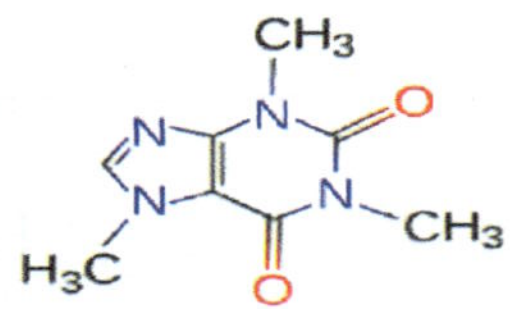 Latex 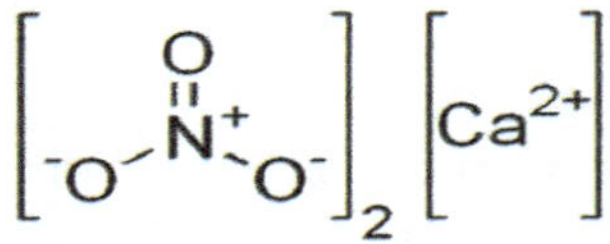 Calcium Nitrate 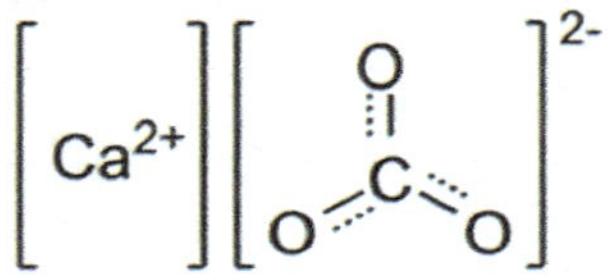 Calcium Carbonate

a)

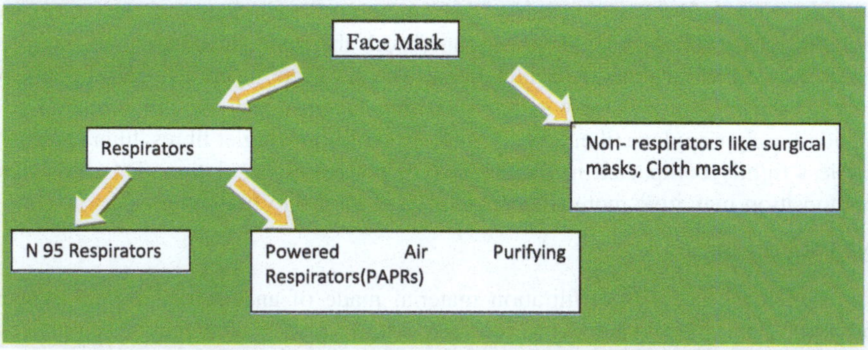

Fig. 2 Various types of **face mask**

Consequently, the utilization of surgical masks by medical personnel is completely common. Nevertheless, surgical masks are not planned for the utilization of preserved healthcare workers from novel diseases. They are mostly outlined to preserve sufferers from whooping cough and discharging of infections from healthcare workers. In this manner, respirators are better as respiratory PPE, principally in a healthcare atmosphere that suppresses novel infections [16]. During the twentieth century, surgical masks were mostly recyclable and produced from multi-layered cotton gauze. Because of this multi-layered formation, the defensive regulation of such masks was increased.

From the mid-twentieth century, lightweight replaceable masks majorly produced from a thin glass fibre non-woven rug were established in the market as a definitive technique of dissuading environmental microorganisms (e.g. bacteria, fungi, and viruses). Till the 1990s, various kinds of fibres (e.g. cellulose and polypropylene) were used for the production of surgical masks. From an elevated quantity of preservative regulation to low cost, they are polypropylene, polyester–rayon, glass, and cellulose. Presently, glass fibre is hardly ever worn and results in infuriation on the worker's skin. Widely used fibre is the polypropylene since it has the ability of water repellence (water-proof) and gives a soft and suitable touch between the face and mask. Modern surgical masks are mainly comprised of three non-woven fabrics layers—a shell fabric, a filter layer, and a cover web. The deepest cover web has a whirl bond with a non-woven rug and more close to the person's skin. Next is the filter layer which lies in between the shell and the cover web. It is a melt-blown non-woven rug firstly discards the airborne particles which are hazardous, body fluids, and microorganisms. The outermost layer is of shell fabric which is revealed to the atmosphere.

Normally, these respirators comprise four–five non-woven fabric layers. Accordingly, two–three layers of non-woven filters are crammed in between the shell fabric and the cover web by polypropylene. The filter layers are made up of tightly filled with a light thin and insubstantial melt-blown non-woven fabric which is based on polypropylene fibre. Additionally, these filter layers are sometimes made up of wiggler fibres which carry the amount of radiation and the combined polypropylene. These wiggler fibres can absorb the toxic substances and microorganisms with the electrostatic attractions. These effects in an elevated amount of safeguarding regulation for wiggler fibre filter layers which are differentiated into standard polypropylene filter layers. Actually, addition wiggler fibres, filter layers set off less tightly compacted in the absence of protecting regulation. This, less tight composition may give more solace and a good ability to breathing [17].

N95 Respirators

An N95 mask consists of filtration material made of an electrostatic non-woven polypropylene fibre that seals to the face, having a 95% efficiency to supply respiratory prevention and decreases the person's revelation to air particulates, from little flecks aerosols to bigger drops as shown in Fig. 3(i) [18]. These masks have the capacity to act as a barrier of particulates and large droplets of the minimum size of 0.3 μm. The prefix letter "N" denotes "non-oil" which means when there is presence of non-oil-based particulates, then the masks can be used in the workplace. In addition, some of these masks are provided with an optional expiration valve which decreases expiration shield, and hence, it makes easy for respiration [19]. The proper wearing of the N95 respirators ensures that the breathing air is being directed through the filter material. National Institute for Occupational Safety and Health (NIOSH) certified the importance of N-95 respirators or greater, for the prevention of inhalation of infectious particle droplets. Size and the mode of particulate transmission play an important role in deciding whether a respirator is required or not. Time to time there is always a demand for upgraded respirators for safety against suspended particulate matter (SPM), liquid droplets, or aerosol particles. Respirators protect from exposure to airborne particles. Its pore size is 0.3 μm [20]. In hospitals, it prevents from disclosure to living droplets which includes viruses and bacteria. Respirators are outlined to cover the person's face. Masks which accumulate at least 95% of the droplets are at 95 in ratings [21]. The good performance of respirator is decided on the basis of two major factors–firstly, the mask should be capable of catching the full scale of toxic particulates, generally at a broad scale of dimensions (<1 to >100 μm) above a scale of air (approx10–100 L/min). Secondly, seepage must be protected at the borderline of the face and the face piece. Rigorous evidence testimonies (42 CFR Part 84) confirmed by NIOSH.

According to NIOSH tests, "worst case" limits which include

- A sodium chloride (for N-series filters) or a dioctyl phthalate oil (for R- and P-series filters) test aerosol with a mass median aerodynamic diameter particle of about 0.3 μm, which is in the MPPS range for most filters
- Airflow rate of 85 L/min, which represents a moderately high work rate
- Conditioning at 85% relative humidity and 38 °C for 24 h prior to testing

Table 2 Ratings for compatibility with oil-based pesticides which show filter efficacy

Ratings for compatibility with oil-based pesticides	Filter efficacy
N—not suitable for use with oil-based pesticides	95—filters 95% of particles from atmosphere
R—oil resistant up to 8 h	99—filters 99% of particles from atmosphere
P—oil proof	100—filters 99.9% of particles from atmosphere

Table 3 Filter description with resisting activity

Oil resistance	Rating	Description
Not oil resistant	N95	Filters at least 95% of particles
	N99	Filters at least 99% of particles
	N100	Filters at least 99.97% particles
Oil resistant	R95	Filters at least 95% of particles
	R99	Filters at least 99% of a particles
	R100	Filters at least 99.97% of airborne particles
Oil proof	P95	Filters at least 95% of particles
	P99	Filters at least 99% of airborne particles
	P100	Filters at least 99.97% particles

- An initial breathing resistance (resistance to airflow) not exceeding 35 mm water column height pressure and initial exhalation resistance not exceeding 25 mm water column height pressure
- A charge-neutralized aerosol
- Aerosol loading conducted to a minimum of 200 mg, which represents a very high workplace exposure
- The filtering efficiency cannot fall below the certification class level at any time during the NIOSH certification tests (Table 2).

Respirators were designed according to their oil resistance as it was invented for oil mines workers [22] (Table 3).

The current medical filters and masks are made up of filters which are observed "fibrous" in creation and are built from plane, on-woven mats of fine fibres. Various factors that play a role in the filtration capacity of how well the filter collects particles depend on fibre breadth, penetrable (the ratio between fibres and open space) and mask diameter thickness. Fibres that are used in the N95 respirator are very crucial and have special mechanical qualities and specifications [23]. The operating capture or filtration mechanism of N95 masks is basically based on the following principles:

Inertial impaction: The inertial impaction collects the larger particles, as the larger particles have higher size or mass, i.e., inertia due to which they do not follow in the air stream and thus move around a filter fibre.

Interception: When the particles present near the filter fibre, they are intercepted and the phenomenon helps to collect the larger particles.
Diffusion: Due to the continuous hitting of smaller particles with air molecules, they deviate and later take place into proximity with a mask fibre and thus are accountable for assembling small particulates [22, 24].
Electrostatic attraction: This mechanism is independent of particle size. The charge fibre has the capability to attract oppositely charged particles.

Amongst the above operating mechanism, the electrostatic attraction mechanism sets these N95 masks apart from other surgical or homemade face masks.

Ideally, these masks shall be thrown away every time when an infected person encounters which succeeds to droplet causing procedures. It can become wet or visibly dirty; get harmed or disfigure; or not extensively should be a productive device to the face which makes it more difficult for the wearer and then be discarded [25]. It can also be adulterated by blood, breathing or nasal discharge or various body liquids and shall be discarded immediately. Though reuse or routine decontamination of these N95 masks is not recommended as per conventional standards of care, however, the shortages of supply of N95 masks during this global pandemic have urged for its decontamination and reuse to ensure continued availability [26]. Various methods that have shown to be potential to decontaminate these masks include ultraviolet germicidal irradiation (UVGI), vaporous hydrogen peroxide (VHP), and moist heat methods. But before adoption of any sterilizing method, evaluation for the capacity to hold up

1. Purifying procedure
2. Suitable disinfectant
3. Persons protection from FFR must be practised [22, 27].

Lewis et al. above-mentioned article has investigated how the use of N95 has provided comparison with hospital health workers infected during influenza outbreaks.

Respirators with high filtration efficiency are considered to be one of the most important and complicated PPEs to manufacture. As per the standard set by NIOSH, only when a 95% filtration efficacy is achieved, and N95 respirators can be sold by manufacturers. Respirators are made using layers of extruded polypropylene plastic fibres (diameter of 1 μm) on a conveyor, which are then bonded to form a cloth as they cool down. Then a hot calendared needled pre-filtration layer of non-woven fabric which should be thick enough to be shaped into a mask is layered on the above fabric. The safeguarding coating of the non-woven thread protects the entire mask. Finally, the manufacturing of masks is completed and is properly sterilized.

The manufactured masks with every batch pass from a series of test which includes oxygen permeability, flammability and beating repellent, particulate sieving regulation and bacteria filtration efficiency, etc. These are specialized masks which are considered to be one of the most important PPEs to be used during this COVID-19 pandemic.

N95 respirators are mainly made of multiple layers of non-woven polypropylene fabric, having the two outward layers which cover the inside and outside of the mask, made using spun bonding using thermal, chemical, and mechanical techniques [14]. The sieving medium upon the mask is been applied as electrostatic non-woven polypropylene polymer. Spun bonding uses nozzles which blow down the melted threads of polypropylene into layers and build up into cloth on a conveyor belt. These two outward layers having density in the range of 20–50 g/m^2 act as the protective barrier against the wearer's exhalations. The layers formed by spun bonding consist of a thick and stiff pre-filtration layer made up of needled non-woven material and a filtration layer. The outermost layer is formed of or polarized non-woven material or melt-blown electrets, which, in turn, determines the efficiency of filtration. The respirators are then added with straps and metal strips for proper adjustment into the user's nose, which is then finally sterilized before physical use [28].

Powered Air Purifying Respirators (PAPRs)

These are additional complex tools respective of characteristics which differ with respective to the mask, face coveralls, helmet, etc. All the PAPRs nevertheless have a machine boaster with energy restoration pack that is attached with a respiratory pack which pushes the airflow towards face as shown in Fig. 3. Filtration of air is done by the canister which is alike with those filters which are used in the renewable masks. PAPRs may have a firmly suited face cover which is manufactured by using silicone and rubber. On the other hand, it can be an appropriate head casing, frequently manufactured by non-woven polypropylene, often made up of PET or acetate. Another efficient alternative of PAPRs is followed by controlled air purifying respirator (CAPR) [14].

Surgical Masks

Surgical masks are willingly obtainable to medical workers and inexpensive as compared to respirators. The FDA-cleared surgical masks are also of great

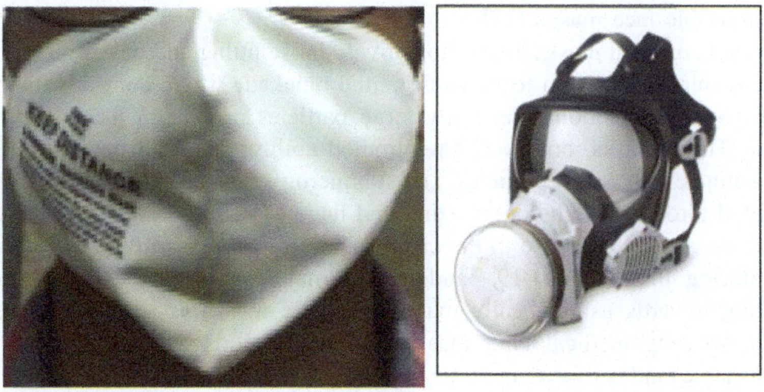

Fig. 3 N95 respirator and PAPR

importance which is planned from the prevention from splashing and spraying which are performed during revelations that are predicted, which includes clinical course of actions, and are highly recommended to be reserved for the healthcare professionals. There are rigorous standards for the evaluation of the efficacy of the surgical masks as personal protective equipment (PPE) used in healthcare settings to check the ability of the masks to protect the wearer from conterminous particles.

The design of these surgical masks usually consists of three-ply material and is generally used to shed potential microorganisms present in infectious airborne and aerosol liquid droplets released from the wearer's mouth and nose. The surgical face mask is generally produced using woven, non-woven, and knitted fabric forming technology [29]. These filters generally consist of one layer of polymeric substance which on each side adjoins the covering of non-woven substance, making a total of 3–4 layers, made using specialized machinery. The degree of filtration efficiency of surgical masks is attained with a very fine filter layer of textile fibres covered on both sides with conventional non-woven bonded fabrics [14]. These masks are most often manufactured of polypropylene, either 20 or 25 g per square metre (GSM) in density, made using spun-bond technology and melt-blown technology, respectively. Also, other polymeric materials such as polystyrene, polycarbonate, polyethylene, or polyester can be also used to manufacture surgical masks of variable sizes for adults as well as infants on-woven are cheaper to make and can be easily cleaned due to their disposable nature, being efficient at sieving out microbes which includes bacteria and viruses above 1 μm. However, microbial sieving efficiency and air permeability of these masks depend on the fibre, manufacturing process, and the fibre's cross-sectional shape. In addition, non-woven fabrics have advantages over woven fabrics infiltration that includes permissible to excessive air, excessive efficacy to bacterial sieving, and lower production cost [30–32]. Then on-woven polypropylene and polymeric substances are provided from drums to the equipment which divides simultaneously, it also unites ultrasonically. The apparatus joins various parts such as metal strips and ear loops, while the filters are sanitized and packed for dispatching. Besides, non-woven surgical face masks being disposable after using present less risk of contamination than either woven or knitted reusable face masks [14].

However, surgical masks are comparatively loose fitting and have efficiency less than the respirators but can form a substantial blockade which connects the person and the capable infections, generally large particles present in the outside environment. These masks, however, have limited ability or do not have any filter to block or inhale very small particles, i.e., submicron-sized airborne particles that get transmitted through coughs or sneezing and have to be discarded after every use.

Cloth masks: In response to the critical shortage of N95 respirators or surgical masks during this COVID-19 pandemic, a major mass of the population are mobilizing towards using locally made cloth face masks as shown in Fig. 4. In addition, wearing medical N95 masks for long periods of time can feel a bit uncomfortable and suffocating, thus, breathable cloth masks are a simple, sustainable, and economic alternative to surgical masks as a means of controlling SARS-COV-2 for the general public masses. These masks made of softer fabric can

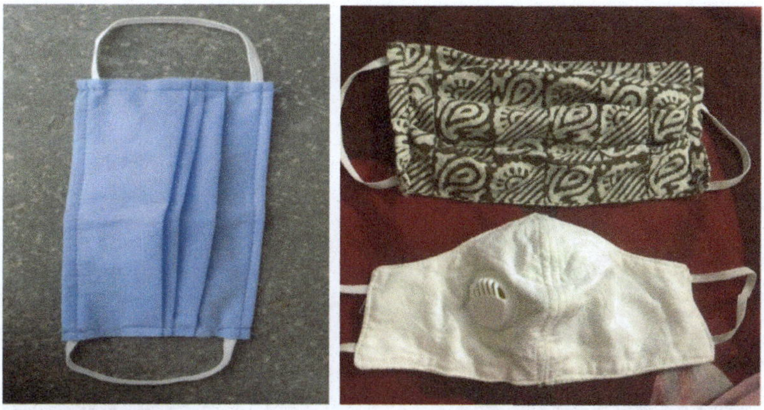

Fig. 4 Surgical mask and cotton cloth mask

be easily made or manufactured at home that can be reused after washing and can be a better option. The cloth masks can be prepared using various types of materials including paper or cloth, but cotton is the most preferred. Though experts agree that cloth face masks absolutely do not alone prevent the spread of COVID-19, wearing a cloth mask will help prevent the spread of droplets that the wearer is emitting and also helps to reduce the chance of infecting others. The fabric of the homemade masks and also the face fitting affect the efficacy of the masks [33].

The universal use of face masks as a means of the source to control the COVID-19 pandemic is strongly advisable. Though homemade face masks cannot prevent the spread of coronavirus, at least cloth masks are efficient as compared to no covering on the face, thus, in turn, reducing the risk of infection. The CDC recommends the easy, effective, and bearable fibres to use at home for covering the face and also has recommended laundering the homemade cloth masks regularly depending on use. Overall, cotton masks with high amount of thread natural silk and chiffon have been found to be performed well. Wearing a mask is the most important habit we can practice to protect ourselves and the communities we live in until a vaccine is developed.

4.2 Dermal PPE

4.2.1 Face Shields

These are the parts of the PPE kits that have been used in healthcare settings and recently became a staple for medical personnel who are in the frontline treating COVID-19 infected patients as shown in Fig. 5. A face shield is simply a curved transparent plastic or Plexiglas panel that can be worn over the face to prevent transmissions of the SARS-CoV-2 coronavirus. Generally, these are not used as

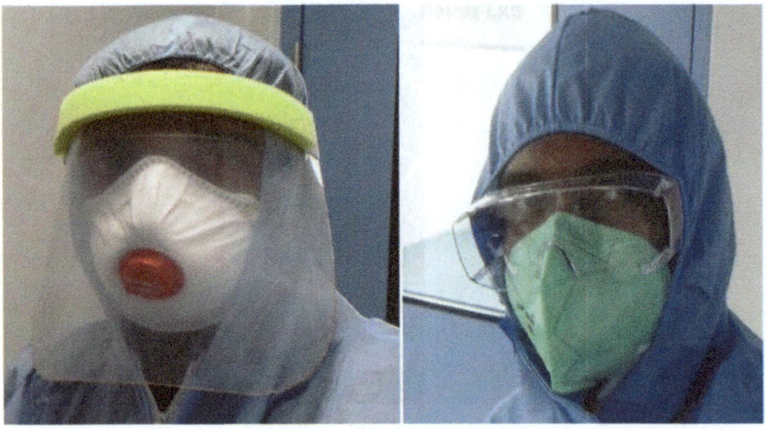

Fig. 5 Face shield and goggle

solitary face/eye protection and are worn in conjunction with other perspective equipment such as masks or respirators, thus blocking infectious droplets and sprays from reaching the face and also reducing the potential for autoinoculation by preventing the health workers from touching their faces frequently. The coverage that face shields offer is ideal since they extend down from the forehead; shields protect the eyes as well as the nose and mouth from the transmission of the contagious infection [34]. The advantage of the face shields is their longevity as they can be well worn for an unlimited time, they can be simply cleaned later every use, comfortable to wear the person from affecting the face, and most eminently, it blocks the entrance of virus from mouth, nose, and eyes. The face shield model(s) to be chosen for appropriate situations will depend upon the circumstances of exposure. In order to be most effective in stopping the viral spread, they should extend below the chin and its width should also be sufficient to cover the ears. In addition, for improved protection there should not be any exposed gap between the forehead and the shield's headpiece.

Face shields are the easiest type of PPE that can be made and consist mainly of three components, namely a visor, an adjustable or non-adjustable frame, and a suspension system with fully or partially circumferential attachment features of the shield to the wearer's head [35]. The visors can come as reusable, replaceable, and disposable models and are generally manufactured of several plastics, namely polycarbonate, propionate, acetate, polyvinyl chloride, and polyethylene terephthalate glycol (PETG). The visitors are frequently provided anti-glare, anti-fog, anti-static, or other advanced protections for their better longevity. Face shield frames can be made up of either plastics or with metal clip-on. Further, the attached suspension systems can be fully circumferential which includes plastic headbands and pin-lock systems or Velcro; non-adjustable structure that engages simple elastic straps, moulded plastic, and 3D-printed plastic. Face shields can be affordably and quickly produced for distribution and thus should be included as an important part of strategies to safely and significantly reduce the transmission of this deadly coronavirus. Some of the simple face shields are designed for single use while others can be sterilized and reused [36].

4.2.2 Eye protection

Reusable face shields or goggles are advised to be used for the protection of eyes. After every use, they should be sanitized, and the disposed products should be flanged out by safe means. These safety options should be eliminated only after departing from the infected person's unit [14].

Protective goggles are deliberated to protect the person's eyes from influenced dangers such as flying pieces, devices, large chips, and morsels. Health professionals need to make use of eye protection goggles using shields when there is a risk from particles. Non-side protected goggles are not tolerable eye safety from the desired risks. The shape of protective goggles is set up of plastic or metal and shall be shaped with the curative or plan effective-impervious lenses. Side shields can be included in the fixture of protective goggles when in need [37].

4.2.3 Gloves

From the past few decades, a significant establishment took place in the manufacturing of surgical gloves. Currently, surgical gloves are basically made up of various waterproof textile polymers (generally produced from nitrile rubber, latex, neoprene, or vinyl) which prevent health protectors from a close approach with infected fluids. Commonly, these gloves can be described as medical gloves and exam gloves as shown in Fig. 6. Exam gloves are generally greased by cornstarch

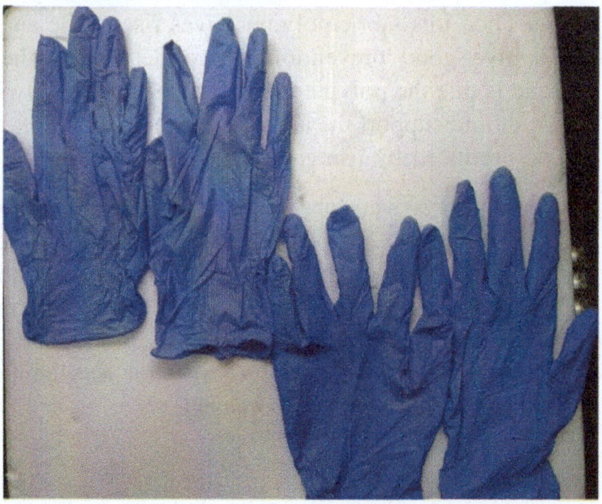

Fig. 6 Gloves

to make them suitable to wear. Medical gloves, although, are not greased, as cornstarch may be taken up by sufferers. Although it is a mandatory deliberation, medical gloves have to be more specific with respect to the person's size to supply the maximum prevention to the sufferers and the medical workers. Non-sterile patient examination gloves including nitrile, natural, rubber, polychloroprene, and vinyl gloves can be used for treating COVID-19 infected patients [38]. Glove restriction depends on the chemical and physical features of the handling stuffs and the kind and time of the work which should be proceeded. This is not necessary that every type of glove will be actually suitable to the skin from the chemical revelations. Chemicals by the time pervade gloves, although they can be carefully used for a particular duration by knowing the features of the gloves such as broadness, pervasion, time and, cost are familiar [39].

4.2.4 Gowns

Apart from hands, the rest of the body parts of medical workers can also be exposed from the liquid. During the nineteenth century, from the prevention of microorganisms, the surgical gowns were invented. Eventually, surgical gowns are white, which represents morality and dignity. Even so, surgical gowns are mostly blue or green in colour, which helps to clear the doctor's vision by refreshing them during surgery. Gowns are stated as "fluid-resistant performance and description of protective at tyres and curtains deliberately for the utilization of the medical means" by the American National Standards Institute/Association of the Advancement of Medical Instrumentation (ANSI/AAMI) PB70:2003. Gowns should completely cover the wearer's body [33, 40].

Thin plastics/paper is used to make the disposable surgical gowns so that they can be reused later. Renewable gowns are often made from natural sources (e.g. cotton) or synthetic source (e.g. polyester fibres). By using the spinning process, these fibres/polymers are then transformed into yarn and then entwined into the fabric. Then this fabric/polymer gives rise to the surgical gown.

To give good prevention and protection to the medical workers, the main demand is that the polymer used for the surgical gown must be water-repellent, and also it should support the air passing easily to it. A water-repellent, airflow polymer can be produced by using:

1. Compactly woven fabrics with a waterproof (fluorochemical or silicone) finish
2. Microporous (<2–3 μm pore size) layers or covering (poly amino acid, polytetrafluoroethylene, polyurethane, acrylics,) on non-woven fabrics of cotton
3. Hydrophilic coverings or layers (such as thermoplastic elastomer based on polyurethane)
4. Sharp or keen polymers (N-tert-butyl acrylamide-ran-acrylamide coated with cotton fabric and shape polymer).

Apart from these basic necessities, a major thing should also be in the demand that there should be no place for the invasion of pathogens in the surgical gowns, since it may cause other infections as well. By using these parameters, the medical workers may get rid of various infections which may be caused by using renewable gowns. For this motive, the disinfectant coats (e.g. metal/silver combined coat, quaternary ammonium compounds finish, N-halamines finish) mostly are done to polymers which are used to prepare the renewable healthcare gowns [41].

Food and Drug Administration (FDA) recognized surgical gowns as Class II medication gadgets and non-sectional gowns as Class I devices which are intended nearly at a dangerous extent (Levels 1–4) and for protection of the user in low or minimal risk isolation situations, respectively. The performance testing of the gowns is very important and is performed using consensus standards by the American Society for Testing and Materials (ASTM) F2407 [33, 42, 43]. For medium to high levels of risks of infection with a large critical zone, it is recommended for the use of ANSI or AAMI PB70 Level 3 or 4 separation robe. While in the surgery or any other levels of exposure, incision robe at levels 1–4 can be preferred and for areas with minimal risk of exposure ANSI/AAMI PB70 Level 1 or 2 gowns can be used.

4.2.5 Coveralls

Coveralls can be worn by health workers as an alternative to gowns having the provision of better protection as shown in Fig. 7. But due to an added layer of insulation, they are more uncomfortable and additionally are often more unfamiliar

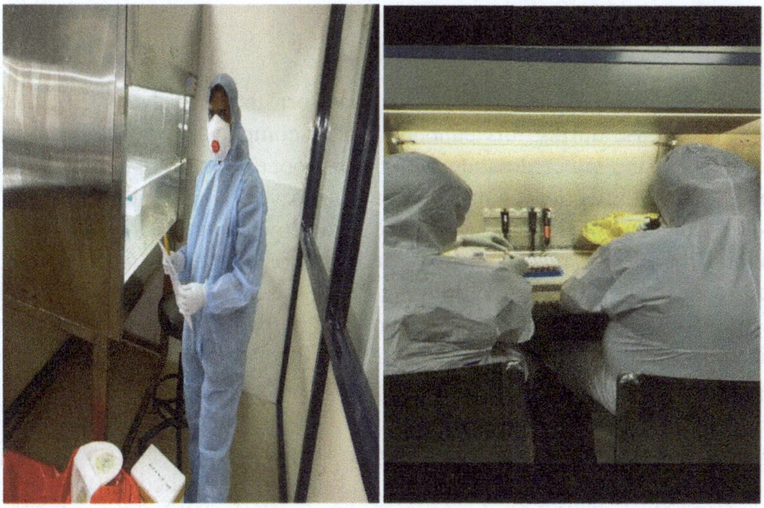

Fig. 7 Coveralls

amongst the healthcare workers, which can thus be risky if the removal of the coveralls is improper. The impermeable fabric for developing coveralls acts as a shielding material between the infectious region and the body parts along with the skin. From the financial point of view, disposable coveralls are a successful substitute cloth defensive outfit. It provides conservation from mould, dust, and numerous different parched morsels and duster menace by which labourers exposed day to day. These replaceable shielding clothes are perfect to use for painting, asbestos or lead subsiding, mould indemnification, food processing, dry chemical application, and a lot more [14].

5 Importance and Value of PPE

The PPE selection depends upon factors like the kinds of subjections leads to splashing/spraying instead of touching, categorization of separated preventions, longevity, and aptness from labour, fitting, etc. The personal protective equipment is important in a number of ways, as it supports in reducing the transmission of highly contagious COVID-19 disease from one infected individual to another.

Also, the lungs of a healthy person get safeguarded while surviving in a contaminated environment. It also protects the eyes of the healthy person from the infections present in the contaminated zone. It further shields the skin against infected materials that may come in contact with the human skin. Due to the use of PPE, mental peace further provides enhanced efficiency in the quality of the working area.

6 Disposing of Contaminated PPE

Though the PPE is the protection aid that is worn to avoid the risk of spreading infection or disease during this pandemic, after completing a task, for example a ward round, visiting infected patients, etc., the proper disposal of all single-use PPE by using standard infection control precautions is very important. The solid waste disposal of all PPEs including facemasks used gloves and other single-use coverings should be ideally placed in dedicated bins or containers with proper lid or covered receptacles. While discarding the PPEs, the major steps should be taken to make sure that the confinements should not hurl in the region where they can infect the wider population. There are certain steps to dispose of the PPEs which depend mostly on the type of infection is participated. For exceedingly threatening materials, a "hazmat" (abbreviated for hazardous materials) team should take care of the PPE and undergo a procedure for tailoring of the correct material. For quality impurities such as lead, the PPE has to be thoroughly washed so that the heavy metals will be discarded. After getting a proper wash, it will be discarded properly to get rid of the danger from the groundwater infection. The most effective way to discard these wastes labelled as infectious PPEs is to burn them as high-temperature destroys the viruses. Other types of used PPE can be land filled or burnt in non-hazardous facilities or recycled. Even the PPE waste handlers should be specifically informed of personal infection control practices including the use of disposable gloves, facemasks, and eye protection to collect the disposed of solid wastes or presumptive SARS-CoV-2 contaminated waste from the specified containers. Containers should be gathered and tightly sealed for transport in a raised-edge or a deep-sided and wheeled cart to prevent leaks and spills during transportation [12].

Each situation and country will have a different set of standards or protocols, which is why it is important for safety managers to keep up to date with the latest Occupational Safety and Health Administration (OSHA) standards in this area. The quarantine centres/wards should be cleaned every two hours, and the waste should be disposed of immediately [44].

Sterilizing, Disinfecting, and Cleaning of PPE

Hydrogen peroxide—In the novel COVID-19 situation, the FDA accepted mechanization progressed by scientific research non-profit Battelle Memorial Institute for the utilization of intensive vapour stage hydrogen peroxide in particular apparatus to disinfect the used N95 respirator masks, as well as different PPE, was worn out by the medical personal. Ethylene oxide is also used to disinfect the personalized protective equipment and different hospitality apparatus which are used by the healthcare workers. Hydrogen peroxide is vigorous in opposition to a broad scope of pathogens which includes the entire microorganism. Economically convenient 3% of hydrogen peroxide solution is strong and productive for plane/surface sanitizing [45]. About 3–6% solution of hydrogen peroxide can sanitize respirators, endoscopes, and polymers. Hydrogen peroxide has been too mentioned in the Environmental Protection Agency's list of sterilizers in opposition to coronavirus.

- Household Cleaners
  Household and trading solutions of bleach may help to sanitize the planes which include renewable apparatus in health centre, pharmaceutical laboratory, physician's workroom from the prevention by the contagious diseases While water and soap are not in stock, the US Centres for Disease Control and Prevention approved the use of hand disinfectants with a congregation of no less than 60% ethanol or 70% isopropyl alcohol to deactivate viruses with the same characteristic features as coronavirus.
- Environmental Protection Agency (EPA) permitted List of Sanitizers
  The American Chemistry Council's Centre for Biocide Chemistries arise recorded outcomes recommended by the Environmental Protection Act (EPA) to use in the opposition to viruses like the SARS-CoV-2, the source of the pandemic COVID-19. EPA's records for list of anti-microbial outcomes which can be used for COVID-19 can be identified [46].

7 Annual Procurement (Demand) for PPE Through UNICEF of PPE

As the COVID-19 has spread globally, the requirement for PPEs has reached extraordinary high and thus the governments have sought to prepare and make available the same to the people. Further, the importance and value of PPE can be accessed from the data available by UNICEF wherein they claimed to supply following PPE items, namely

- Face shield, smog-repellent, face cover
- Goggles, shielding, divergent air blower
- Masking, non-returnable, citizen's use
- High sieving masks, N95/FFP2, FFP2/N95, no nozzle, aseptic
- Mask, resectional, rope belt, non-returnable, type IIR,
- Cap, resectional, puffy, non-fabricated
- Slacks, resectional, fabricated
- Robe, resectional, fabricated
- Robe, resectional, aseptic, non-fabricated
- Overall, shielding, flexible, non-returnable
- Overall, shielding, flexible, recyclable
- Overall, shielding, type 6b, Cat III
- Gloves, non-returnable, w/o granulate, nitrile
- Gloves, dreadful, nitrile/latex
- Gloves, non-returnable, nitrile, w/o granulate
- Boots, recyclable, PVC/latex, pair
- Boot sheath, slip-resistant, stretchable.

During the last four months, i.e., February–May, the supply of PPE kits were increased as depicted in Fig. 8. In the month of April, maximum PPE kits have been supplied contracted through UNICEF [47].

The yearly acquisition (ultimatum) for Personal Protective Equipment via UNICEF from 2017 to 2020 has been shown in figure.

According to Figs. 8 and 9, it is understood that the basic need for humans is to use the face mask, as per the pandemic guidelines, and it became mandatory to use the mask if a person is outside or exposed directly to the environment. The demand and supply for the face mask were very high in the month of April due to the increasing COVID-19 cases. As per the current situation, still, the demand for the face mask is much more as compared to the other PPEs, and hence, the supply for the respective is high.

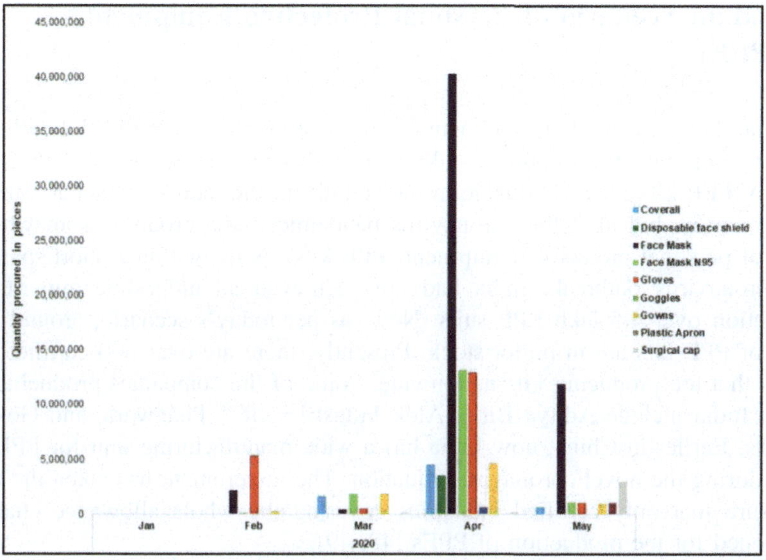

Fig. 8 Supply contracted through UNICEF. *Source* January–May 2020 https://www.unicef.org/supply/stories/covid-19-impact-assessment-and-outlook-personal-protective-equipment

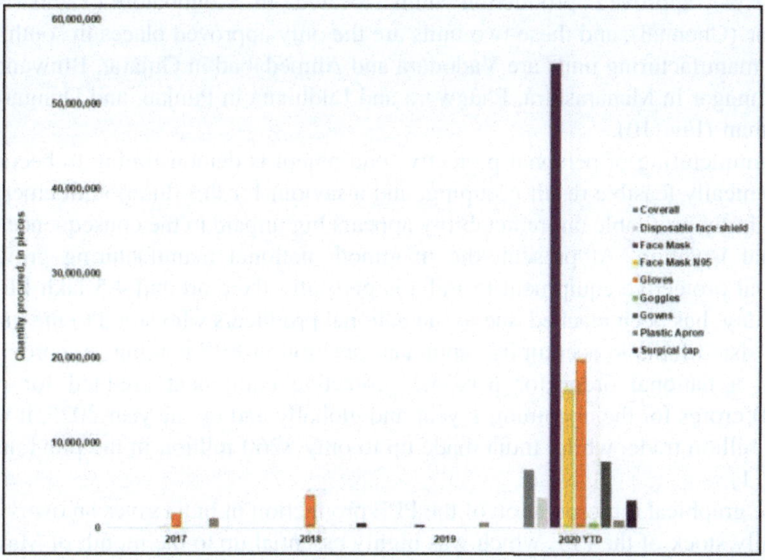

Fig. 9 Annual procurement (demand) for PPE through UNICEF between 2017 and 2020 year to date. *Source* YTD https://www.unicef.org/supply/stories/covid-19-impact-assessment-and-outlook-personal-protective-equipment

8 Indian Scenario of Personal Protective Equipment's (PPE)

In India, there was no domestic manufacturing of even a single PPE kit earlier and all were imported from countries like China, Russia, and Spain, etc. About 2.75 lakhs of PPE kits were obtainable in the country in the month of January, that too was imported, but after the coronavirus pandemic, India produces somewhat 2.6 lakhs of personal protective equipment (PPE kits). Now, within a short span after the coronavirus outbreak, India had now achieved an unfeasible aim of daily production over 4.5 lakh PPE suits. Now, as per today's scenario, around 15.96 lakhs of PPE kits are in buffer stock. Presently, there are over 600 certified companies that are producing kits nationwide. Some of the companies producing PPE kits in India include Aditya Birla, Alok Industries, JCT Phagwara, and Gokaldas Exports. Earlier in China, now India has a wide manufacturing unit for PPE coveralls during the novel coronavirus situation. The government has taken the action to ensure that only certified industries covering the whole allowance chain are sanctioned for the production of PPEs [48, 49].

In India, Bangalore is the PPE hub as it serves 50% of the daily PPE kit production in the nation. Apart from Bangalore, Tamil Nadu, Gujarat, Punjab, Maharashtra, Rajasthan, Kolkata, Delhi, Noida, and Gurugram are the places where PPE kits are being manufactured. The Ministry of Health and Family Welfare (MoHFW) approved production units located in Coimbatore (Tamil Nadu), Tirupur (Chennai), and these two units are the only approved places in south India. Other manufacturing units are Vadodara and Ahmedabad in Gujarat, Bhiwandi and Kusumnagar in Maharashtra, Phagwara and Ludhiana in Punjab, and Dungarpur in Rajasthan (Fig. 10).

Manufacturing of personal protective equipment is demonstrating to become an economically feasible result grouping, and a saviour for this duration of emergency accordingly profitable unpredictability appears big unpaid to the consequence of the national isolation. At present, the mammoth national manufacturing growth of personal protective equipment in India is presently fixed around 4.5 lakh PPE kits every day, has been reached due to the national producers who stood to the instance and assisted India to accomplish abundant position in PPE making. According to a report, a national order for personal protective equipment credited for rupees 10,000 crores for the upcoming 1 year and globally and by the year 2025, it will be a $60 billion trade, while, India made up to only $260 million in the previous year (Fig. 11).

The graphical representation of the PPE production in India gives an overview of the daily stock of the PPE which was highly essential up to the month of May. The graph shows the rapid increase in the production of PPE kits. As the month of May was the peak point for the coronavirus cases, there was an instant need for the PPEs which gives a shielding effect regarding the pandemic disease. As the graph suggests, there was no production of PPE kits in the month of March as these kits were being imported from the other countries. But depending on the increased cases, the

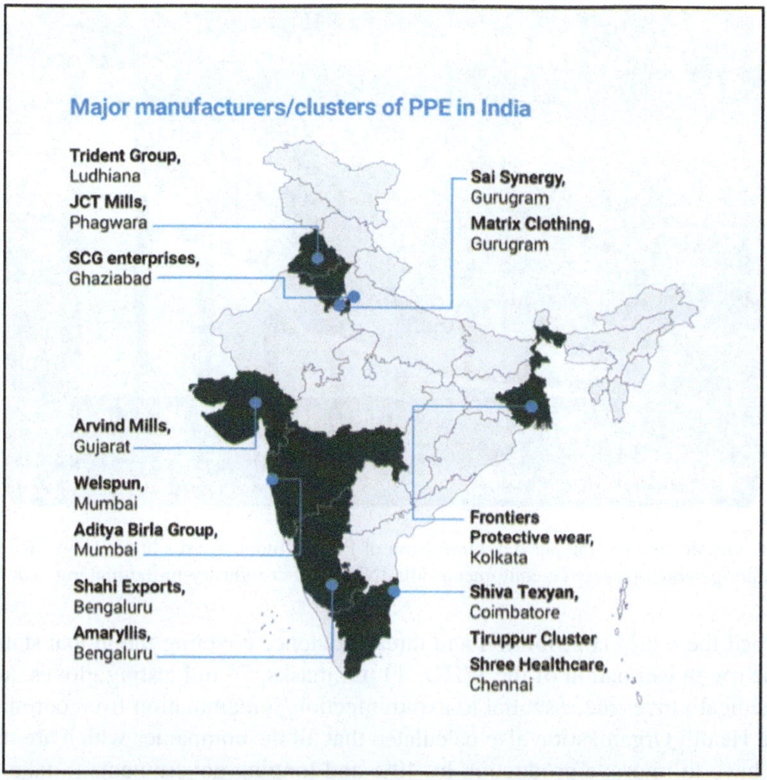

Fig. 10 Major manufacturers/clusters of PPE in India. *Source* https://www.investindia.gov.in/siru/personal-protective-equipment-india-INR-7000-cr-industry-in-the-making [10]

government took a decision to manufacture the PPE kits in the nation. Approx. 4 lakhs of PPE kits were manufactured in the month of March depending upon a daily basis. And this is how India became the second-largest country in the world for the manufacturing of the PPE kits.

9 World Scenario of Personal Protective Equipment (PPE)

Due to the rapid increase in the coronavirus infections, the Asia-Pacific region has gone through an unpredicted inclination in the conditions for PPE kits. This region reports the wide-reaching contamination because of which PPE kits have gained more importance, value, and use especially for battle line labourers, and employees operating in different companies. Besides, gush request, partly fixed with dread purchase, stockpile, and misapply of personal protective equipment (PPE), has

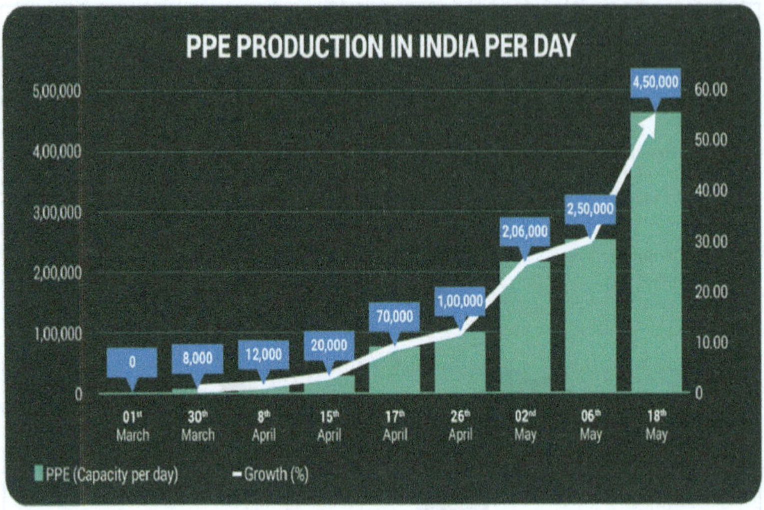

Fig. 11 Graph showing the per day production of PPE in India. *Source* https://www.investindia.gov.in/siru/personal-protective-equipment-india-INR-7000-cr-industry-in-the-making [10]

disturbed the world contribution and threat existence covering the global status. As per the rough estimation of the WHO, 89 mil masks, 76 mil testing gloves, and 1.6 mil medical gloves are essential to avoid infection/contamination from coronavirus. World Health Organization also calculated that all the companies which are making PPEs have to improve production by 40% and longing governments to take action rapidly to uplift stores and are anticipating charging the PPE stock in a small time span. The PPE kits are also globally utilized by the establishment of employees due to the dangerous places and atmosphere. China is an important vendor for the personal protective equipment stock owing to the broad enlargement of its railways. Furthermore, the Chinese expenditure on railways is awaited to increase by about 6% every year to USD 125 billion in 2020 for the establishment of a fast-moving rail web [50].

10 Future Perspective and Key Market Trends of Personal Protective Equipment (PPE)

The PPE market is looking forward to increasing at a compound annual growth rate (CAGR) of 7.8% above the augur duration 2020–2025. The growing figures of coronavirus sufferers, besides, the increase in the commercial consciousness of worker conservation at the organizational level, are the crucial elements that operate the wide scope utilization of various PPE. In addition, the enlargement of the greater and upgraded status of medicines in laboratories has inclined the specification of PPE in the medical section.

Growing expenditure in experimentation and expansion of immunization in opposition to contagious or global diseases is awaited to power the stipulation for the market. Moreover, it saves the medical workers from infectious disease vulnerability in the organization, such as operation theatres and ICUs, research laboratories, which is awaited to occur in the future. Further, the Occupational Safety and Health Administration (OSHA) also emanates the statute for the organization of welfare and health of the caretakers by disclosing to mycobacterium tuberculosis and blood-borne microorganisms. Nevertheless, by Occupational Safety and Health Administration's General Duty article, personal protective equipment is needed for some potent communicable illness disclosure. Workers should be provided with suitable PPE and make sure that PPE should be disposed of or, if durable, it should be properly repaired, cleaned, and then only it should be reused. Increasing cases of coronavirus have rapidly inclined the orders for PPE mainly face shields, preventive gowns, medical masks, disposable gloves, and preventive goggles, worldwide. It has led to a scarcity in the supply and is dangerous for both patients and caretakers. China is the wide distributor of the essentials needed to fight with the virus and had marketed personal protective equipment that many of it came out to be damaged. In case, Spain had given back 50,000 personal protective equipment to China after finding that they were defective. Also, from China, India imported 170,000 PPE kits that broke down the standard trials as per Indian Standards and was also given back. The USA has also bought the medical contribution, as well as PPE and ventilators, from Russia. Both the countries did not expose the figure of therapeutic contributions that were delivered to the USA. Besides conceding the importance of PPE outside patient care by usual natives to protect oneself from the novel coronavirus, collaborators in the providing links are purchasing present chances to increase the ruthless cost of their results. To embellish out the contribution, the ministry is raising its manufacturing abilities. Mentioning the case of April 2020, US President Donald J. Trump had supplicated the Defence Production Act (DPA) and provided an administrative instruct to General Motors to provide N95 respirator masks and ventilators for the confederate government [50, 51].

The worldwide personal protection equipment was estimated at $52.7 billion in 2019 and is awaited to extend till $92.5 billion by 2025, increasing up to a CAGR of 8.7% in the years 2020–2025 (Fig. 12).

11 COVID-19 Pandemic Market Impact in USA

North America is undergoing industrialization at a widening speed which gives rise to the figure of production protocols and course of action with the small parts owing to which personal protective equipment industries are concentrating on scheming distinctive preservative outfits to make sure best security for employees. As the production section complicated some main and additional procedures for connecting and metal production, employees are often revealed to the atmosphere that can result in project coincidence. As per the Bureau of Labour Statistics (BLS), it

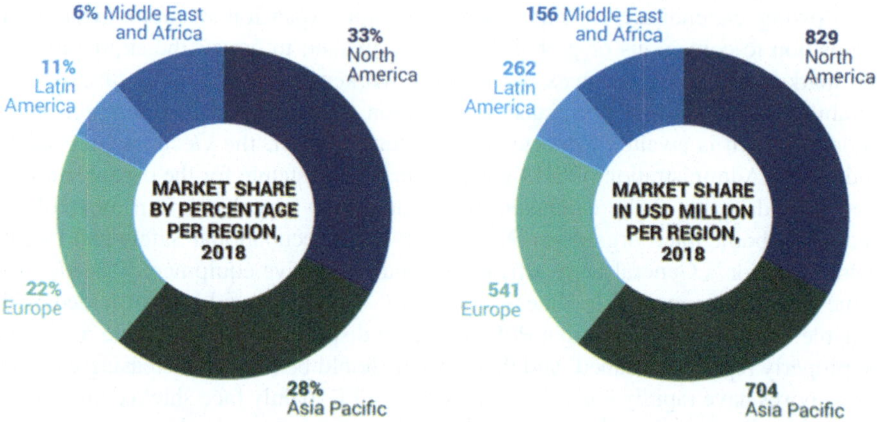

Fig. 12 Global PPE market. *Source* https://www.investindia.gov.in/siru/personal-protective-equipment-india-INR-7000-cr-industry-in-the-making [10]

described 5147 organizations casualties in the USA in 2017. Between these casualties, 887 owing to deadly falls, which is the peak stage described in the 26-year history of the Census of Mortal Work Injuries. Furthermore, by June 2020, USA has the excessive figure of coronavirus sufferers owing to which there is a prong in order for personal protective equipment for caretaker's solicitation in the USA has fascinated many expenditures in the vend. In May 2020, the Department of Defence, coordinated with Department of Health and Human Services and approved a USD 126 million agreement granted by 3M for the elevated manufacturing of 26 million N95 surgical class masks each month in opposition to pandemic situations. Furthermore, during January 2020, the industries so far uphold the manufacturing of respirators and enlarged the world production up to 1.1 billion every year, as well as 35 million N95 masks every month in USA in additionally, in Canada, The Ontario government has spent CAD 200 million in obtaining healthcare products, which includes four million face shields, 100 million surgical masks, and 20 million gowns [51].

12 Future Perspective of Personal Protective Equipment (PPE) Market

- ***COVID-19 Pandemic Market Impact in USA***
  See Fig. 13.
- ***COVID-19 Pandemic Market Impact in World***

  See Fig. 14.

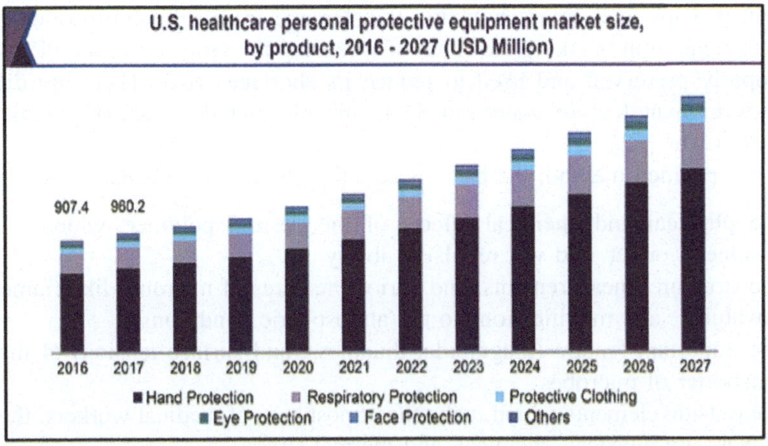

Fig. 13 Healthcare personal protective equipment market size in USA. *Source* Healthcare personal protective equipment market size, share and trends analysis report by product (respiratory protection, hand protection), by end use, by region, and segment forecasts, 2020–2027 [11]

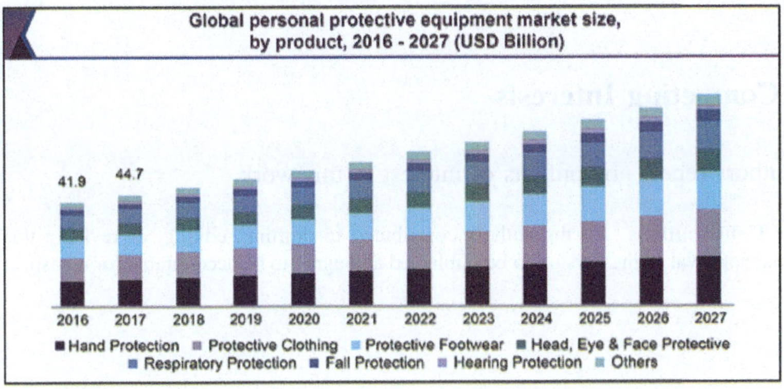

Fig. 14 Global personal protective equipment market size, by product, 2016–2027. *Source* Healthcare personal protective equipment market size, share and trends analysis report by product (respiratory protection, hand protection), by end use, by region, and segment forecasts, 2020–2027 [51]

13 Summary

The present review reveals the importance and value of PPEs as radiation shielding material against the pandemic coronavirus. It focused on the use and importance of PPEs which helps in reducing the transmission of COVID-19 infection and thus protects the end-users from getting infected. Also, the purpose and role of PPE are non-replaceable and most important in this global crucial era of COVID-19, wherein it helps to decrease infection transference from sufferers to other people and thus helping in breaking the chain of spreading the virus. Also, the PPE should be properly preserved and used to reduce its shortage crisis. There are different methods to manufacture water-repellent, airflow, and disinfectant polymers for surgical gowns [52].

For a specified method, the basic necessities should be considered as follows:

1. The physical and chemical effects of the desired polymer, which includes broadness, outlet, and wet repulsive ability
2. The structure, measurements, and various features of microbes like framework, movability, and modifications to the atmospheric conditions
3. The important feature (magnitude, thickness, and surface tension) of the fluid transporter of microbes
4. The outside elements which make the atmosphere of medical workers, the most relevant are physical, chemical, and thermal stress.

PPE is used to be an important part for safety purposes for everyone. It helps in protecting from the direct exposure of the contaminant. Prior to use, the PPE kits must be checked whether it is defective or not. It is also mandatory to dispose or clean it after every use so that the person will be protected from the infection [39].

14 Competing Interests

The authors report no conflicts of interest in this work.

Author Contributions All the authors contributed to drafting, editing, or revising the article, gave final approval of the version to be published and agree to be accountable for all aspects of the work.

References

1. Rowan NJ, Laffey JG (2020) Challenges and solutions for addressing critical shortage of supply chain for personal and protective equipment (PPE) arising from coronavirus disease (COVID19) pandemic–case study from the Republic of Ireland. Sci Total Environ. 138532
2. https://www.dailymail.co.uk/
3. https://cen.acs.org/index.html
4. http://www.cshl.edu/
5. Fish JT, Stout RN, Wallace E (2010) Practical crime scene investigations for hot zones. CRC Press
6. Casanova L, Rutala WA, Weber DJ, Sobsey MD (2010) Coronavirus survival on healthcare personal protective equipment. Infect Control Hosp Epidemiol 31(5):560–561
7. Balkhyour MA, Ahmad I, Rehan M (2019) Assessment of personal protective equipment use and occupational exposures in small industries in Jeddah: health implications for workers. Saudi J Biol Sci 26(4):653–659

8. Bajwa SJ, Sarna R, Bawa C, Mehdiratta L (2020) Peri-operative and critical care concerns in coronavirus pandemic. Indian J Anaesth 64(4):267
9. Cook TM (2020) Personal protective equipment during the coronavirus disease (COVID) 2019 pandemic–a narrative review. Anaesthesia
10. https://onlinelibrary.wiley.com/
11. https://www.investindia.gov.in
12. https://mafiadoc.com/
13. Jain S, Yadav Lamba B, Kumar S, Singh D (2020) Strategy for repurposing of disposed PPE kits by production of biofuel: pressing priority amidst COVID-19 pandemic. Biofuels 1–5
14. Advincula RC, Dizon JRC, Chen Q, Niu I, Chung J, Kilpatrick L, Newman R (2020) Additive manufacturing for COVID-19: devices, materials, prospects and challenges. MRS Communications
15. https://www.thomasnet.com/network/
16. https://www.safety.duke.edu.com/
17. https://www.technicaltextile.net/
18. https://www.honeywell.com/en-us
19. https://honeywellconsumerstore.com/
20. Huang SH, Chen CW, Kuo YM, Lai CY, McKay R, Chen CC (2012) Factors affecting filter penetration and quality factor of particulate respirators. Aerosol Air Qual Res 13(1):162–171
21. https://www.ccohs.ca/
22. https://www.cdc.gov/
23. http://ps-survival.com/PS/index.htm
24. Prasetyo A, Adi Rahardja A, Tsuroya Azzahro D, Pawitra Miranti I, Saraswati I, Nur Kholis F (2019) Nephrolepis exaltata herbal mask increases nasal IgA levels and pulmonary function in textile factory workers. Adv Prev Med 2019
25. Rodriguez-Martinez CE, Sossa-Briceño MP, Cortés-Luna JA (2020) Decontamination and reuse of N95 filtering facemask respirators: a systematic review of the literature. Am J Infect Control
26. De Perio MA, Dowell CH, Delaney LJ, Radonovich LJ, Kuhar DT, Gupta N, Patel A, Pillai SK, D'Alessandro M (2020) Strategies for optimizing the supply of N95 filtering facepiece respirators during the coronavirus disease 2019 (COVID-19) pandemic. Disaster Med Public Health Prep 14(5):658–669
27. Umer FA, Haji Z, Zafar KA (2020) Role of respirators in controlling the spread of novel coronavirus (Covid-19) among dental health care providers: a review. Int Endod J
28. https://www.honeywellstore.com/
29. http://www.teamtsi.com/
30. https://dost.gov.ph/
31. https://business.thomasnet.com/about
32. https://www.slideshare.net/
33. https://medium.com/
34. https://www.pulmonologyadvisor.com/
35. http://webhosting.kify.com/
36. Roberge RJ (2016) Face shields for infection control: a review. J Occup Environ Hyg 13 (4):235–242
37. https://extension.wvu.edu/
38. https://ehs.research.uiowa.edu/
39. https://www.resultsdirect.com/home
40. Viscusi DJ, Bergman MS, Eimer BC, Shaffer RE (2009) Evaluation of five decontamination methods for filtering facepiece respirators. Ann Occup Hyg 53(8):815–827
41. https://journals.lww.com/pages/default.aspx
42. https://www.temple.edu/research
43. https://www.chemicalsafetyfacts.org/chemistry-context/
44. https://www.creativesafetysupply.com/qa/ppe/what-is-the-proper-way-to-dispose-of-ppe
45. https://www.unicef.org/research-and-reports

46. https://timesofindia.indiatimes.com/india/from-zero-india-now-produces-around-2-lakh-ppe-kits-per-day/articleshow/75556879.cms
47. http://www.globenewswire.com/Index
48. Priyadarshini R, Jafrin L, Aravinthan A, Sivagnanam G (2020) Rationing PPEs during a pandemic: the COVID-19 scenario. Res Soc Adm Pharm
49. https://www.grandviewresearch.com/
50. https://www.ijbts-journal.com/
51. https://covid19biblio.com/keyword-co-occurrence/
52. https://www.researchsquare.com/coronavirus

Chapter 4
Exploration of Inorganic Materials with Antiviral Properties

Sushree Pattnaik, Balamati Chaudhury, and Mamata Mohapatra

1 Introduction

The recent pandemic has led to worldwide requirement for efficient detection and therapies reducing its effect. There is availability of materials which are reported to be efficient because of their physicochemical properties flexible chemical functionalization offering multiple ways to handle the urgent crisis. It has been reported using multidisciplinary perception around various fields like virology, medicine, biology etc. We sketch out the use of various procedures or approaches viable to fight against recent outbreak, also including future pandemics and infectious diseases. As per the studies done to identify the life cycle of virus, researchers can foresee the procedures where using nanotechnology they can combat the disease. Figure 1 shows the process of infection of host cell by virus. The nanoparticles propose substitutes for the existing disinfection protocols and their inherent anti-pathogenic properties and having potential in inactivation of viruses, bacteria, fungi etc. via photo thermal process or by generation of reactive halogen, oxygen and nitrogen species. The drugs designed using nanotechnology reported to have potential to inactivate SARS-CoV-2 virus in patients. They could also be utilized for drug delivery to pulmonary system for restricting the interactions between ACE 2 receptors and viral S protein. The concept of "Nano-immunity by design" will be utilized for designing drugs for immune modulation via their stimulation or suppression of responses and will be helpful for vaccine development. Nanotechnology

S. Pattnaik (✉) · M. Mohapatra
CSIR-Institute of Minerals and Materials Technology, Bhubaneswar 751013, India
e-mail: mamata@immt.res.in

S. Pattnaik · B. Chaudhury · M. Mohapatra
Academy of Scientific and Innovative Research (AcSIR), Ghaziabad, Uttar Pradesh 201002, India

B. Chaudhury
Centre for Electromagnetics, CSIR-NAL, Bangalore, India

M. Mohapatra et al. (eds.), *COVID-19 Pandemic*, Materials Horizons: From Nature to Nanomaterials, https://doi.org/10.1007/978-981-16-4372-9_4

helps in developing simple and cheaper assays and biomarkers to monitor SARS-CoV-2. Nanotechnology is quite important in fighting against COVID-19 and future pandemic outbreaks. The progress of antiviral treatments usually need years before they are made extensively available [1] as there are a variety of regulatory stages needed for establishment of their safety and efficiency [2]. Due to the mutation of SARS-CoV-2, the target specific viral drugs might change which leads to resisting the therapy and medication which has already been observed, whilst treating other viral diseases. Reportedly, there has been an increasing demand for novel and all-purpose antiviral compounds which are less resisting and could be utilized for a variety of viruses which includes newly originated viruses [3–5]. Such kinds of therapies are recommended till more refined, and target specific drugs and vaccines are available for new viruses. Nanotechnology has been reported to propose a number of procedures for combating viruses outside and inside the host and many of them are successful in preclinical studies for countering the viral pathogens like HIV, human papilloma virus, herpes simplex and respiratory viruses [3–6].

The approaches are mainly focused on developing the inhibitors [7, 8]. An extremely preserved part of viruses is the attachment ligand (VAL). In case of the respiratory viruses, [9] VAL has been reported to target heparan sulphate proteoglycans (HSPG) [10] or sialic acids (SA) [11]. HSPG and SA mimics have been reported to show in vitro skills to attach to viruses, restricting their contact with the cell membranes [12–14]. The perspective of nano medicine has led to the progress of the nanomaterials which ranges from polymers [15] to dendrimers, [16] oligomers, NPs, [17] liposomes, [18] and small molecules [19]. Clinical translation has been reported to be hindered when diluted and they tend to lose their efficiency when the virus compound complex dissociates letting the virus free to replicate again. Lately, it has been reported that the limitations could be eradicated by preparing NPs which after binding, restricts the viral infection by destructing the virion, which leads to all-purpose antiviral drugs [20]. The focus is mainly on a specific drug for SARS-CoV-2, which would be a good entry inhibitor capable of

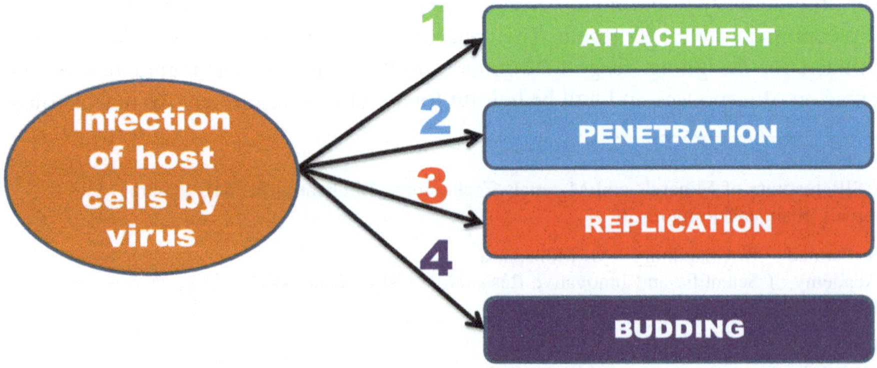

Fig. 1 This figure illustrates infection process of the host cells by virus

blocking the S spike protein relation with that of cellular ACE2 receptor [21–24]. Apart from the specific approach, it is vital that novel, efficient antivirals are reported to be based on compounds which show very little or almost negligible toxicity profiles, as the patients would be administered those drugs for extended time period and it leads to weakening of body. Due to these reasons, the clearance mechanisms are considered thoroughly, whilst designing these antiviral drugs. An illustration of the procedure is the new redesign of wide utilization antiviral NPs into evenly efficient customized cyclodextrins [25].

2 Inorganic Materials with Antiviral Properties

2.1 Nanoparticles as Potential Antiviral Candidates

Its evolution due to which viruses have different molecular mechanisms to enter into a cell, helping them in survival for longer period, activation, or replication at various levels [26]. They are reported to have the ability of transferring genes efficiently which led to developing viral vectors that are not infectious for gene therapy [27–29]. Trials are being made for enhancing the safety of the viral vectors. More studies are reportedly being carried out by the researchers in nano medicine for making systems capable of replicating the gene transfer and the high infectivity of those vectors. Elucidating the molecular mechanisms behind these reported vectors, researchers are preparing delivery systems for treatment in various fields including therapies and medicines [30, 31]. Nanotechnology is reportedly using virology to develop as well as combat the viruses. One of the main causes of mortality these days worldwide has been viral infections and also the reason for loss of economy [32, 33]. The treatment procedures include vaccination and therapies which are only reported to target the life cycle of virus. Figure 2 shows the interacting stages of nanoparticles with viruses. Viruses, have believed to evolve under pressures, have become more resistant towards drugs due to which there is the need of new drugs. Nano medicine is one of the budding areas of nanotechnology with broad range of utilizations in pharma and diagnosis [34, 35]. As per reports, metal nanoparticles are regarded as potential drug transport agents for specific targets in body, these materials could be optimized as drug delivery systems [36]. Since primeval time noble metals are reported to be therapeutic agents in the field of medicine. Predominantly, Ag, Au and Pt nanoparticles are reported to have the stability to withstand in an intracellular [37, 38]. Small-sized stable nanoparticles have been reported to show advantage that easily relates with the bio-molecules present at surface and inside the cells playing an important part in the biomedical applications of diagnosis and treatments.

Silver is reported to have antibacterial properties [39] and recently studies show the use of its antiviral and immune-modulatory properties as nanoparticles [40, 41].

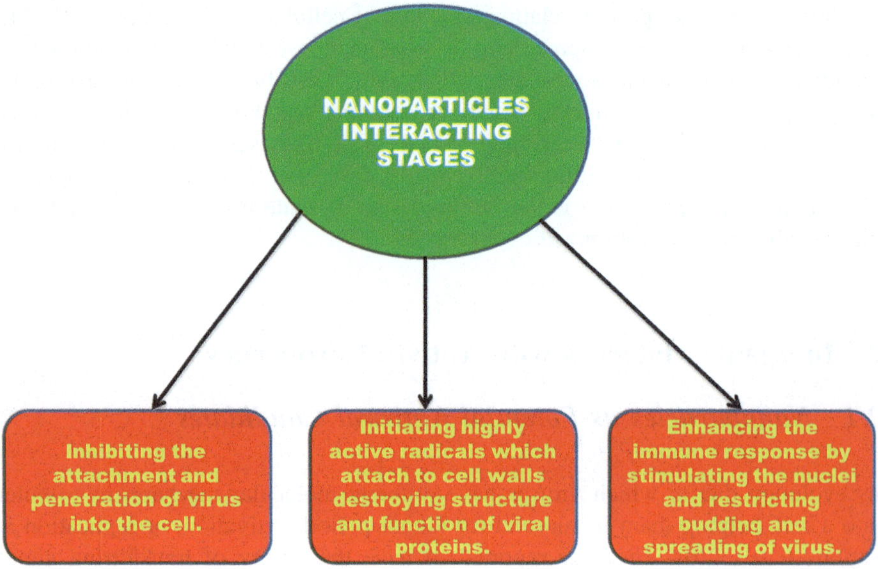

Fig. 2 This figure illustrates interacting stages of nanoparticles

Morris and co-worker [42] have reported the in vivo antiviral activity of Ag NPs (RSV) infection.

Nanoparticles of noble metals are reported as potential candidates with both the antiviral and antibacterial properties as drug delivery agent to target and reducing the side effects. It has been reported that quantum and classical atomistic molecular dynamics computational way to reveal adsorption properties of hydroxychloroquine on the noble metal nanoparticles. Adsorption energy reported for hydroxychloroquine is less than 30 kcal mol^{-1} and its (non) perturbative properties on the plasmonic absorption spectra of silver and gold nanoparticles characterized with time-dependent density functional theory. The reports of size effects and compositions of nanoparticles have been obtained for hydroxychloroquine and chloroquine stated as candidates for drug delivery. The modelling so reported helped researchers for competent and secure therapeutics.

2.1.1 Metal-Based Nanomaterials as Antiviral Materials

The metal-based nanoparticles were reported to possess distinctive physicochemical properties attributed to their small size and surface area that allowed them to interact with viruses. A range of metal and metal oxide NPs has been reported as antiviral agents [40]. Figure 3 depicts some of the metal-based NPs utilized due to their antiviral properties.

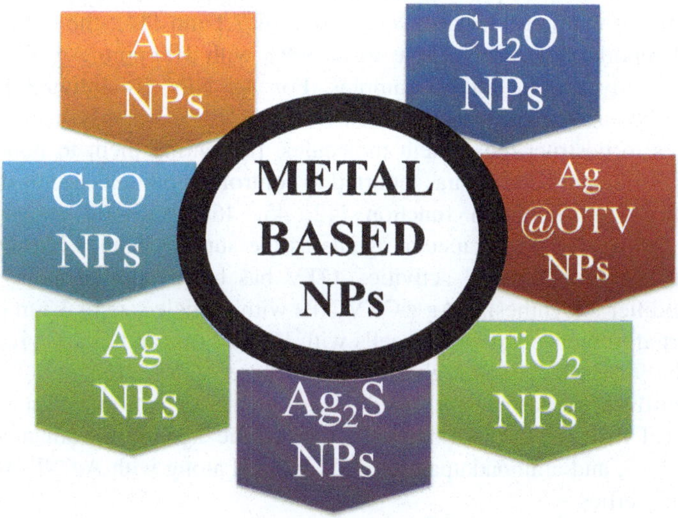

Fig. 3 This figure illustrates some metal-based nanoparticles with antiviral properties

Silver-Based Antiviral Nanoparticles

It has been reported silver metal, and its derivative have anti-microbial properties and also have notable anti-pathogen activity. Ag NPs are reported to interact with the viruses inhibiting their attachment and penetration to the host cells. The average particle size of Ag NPs is an important factor that affects its antiviral ability. Ag NPs with particle size 33 nm has been reported to be synthesized using chemical reduction procedure controls herpes (HSV-2) infection in mice efficiently by restricting the bond of virus with the host [43]. These are reported not to show any toxicity and pro-inflammatory cases. The comparison of various types of AgNPs based on their preparation and utilization is given in Table 1.

Table 1 Comparison of various types of Ag NPs

S. No.	Types	Particle size (nm)	Preparation	Applications	References
1	Ag NPs	33	Chemical reduction	Effective against HSV-2	[43]
2	Ag NPs	7.1	Electrochemical method	Cell survival rate 98%	[44]
3	Ag@OTV	3	OTV acts as surface modifier	Effective against H1N1 virus Cell survival rate 90%	[47]
4	Ag_2S NPs	5	Prepared using glutathione	Inhibits PEDV more than 99%	[48]

Ag NPs with smaller particle size has been reported to be synthesized using electrochemical method with an average size of 7.1 nm [44], the cultural studies performed reports cell survival rate to be 98% with 100 ppm Ag NPs with cell viability of only 2% in control samples. For Ag NPs, its antiviral function is reported to be easily related to the fact that these NPs can easily interact with the polioviruses to destruct the protein molecules, preventing them to bond with the host cells. Surfactant addition has reported to control the particle size of the Ag NPs improving its anti-infection function [42, 45, 46]. Antiviral activity can be improved by the use of therapeutic agents as the surface ligands like Oseltamivir (OTV) an agent for antiviral activities. OTV has been reported to be used as a surface modifier to synthesize Ag@OTV NPs with particle size of 3 nm [47]. It has been reported to be used to culture cells with H1N1 virus and the survival rate was found to be 90% which was high than that of bare AGMPs (65%).

The improvement has been reported due to synergistic anti-infection effect of Ag NPs and OTV ligands. Other reported therapeutic agents are amantadine [49], zanamivir [50], and aminoadamantane [51] utilized along with Ag NPs to boost its antiviral properties.

There are many more compounds of Ag with reported antiviral properties. Ag_2S nanoparticles (Ag_2S NCs) have been reported to have particle size of 5 nm prepared using glutathione which was the capping agent [52]. It has been reported to be used to inhibit porcine epidemic diarrhoea virus (PEDV) more than 99%, and it affects other viruses as well. Other reported silver compounds are silver bis (citrato) germinate [53], $AgNO_3$ [54] and silver acesulfame [55] are efficient anti-virus materials. Ag NPs have been reported to have potential antiviral properties and are efficient against variety of viruses like HIV-1, monkey pox virus, [56] bacteriophages UZ1 and MS2, [57, 58] murine norovirus MNV1, [57, 58] HSV, [59] HBV, [60] and recently, in porcine epidemic diarrhoea virus (PEDV) [48]. Ag NPs antiviral properties have been reported to take place via three different kinds of mechanisms. As per studies first, Ag(0) NPs dissolves and leads to release of some noxious Ag(I) which also includes Ag^+ ions capable of antiviral activity. Ag being a soft metal has quite a strong affinity towards sulphur and therefore has interactions with the thiols in the active sites of enzymes. Ag(I) may interact with surface proteins of viruses or accumulate in host cells and further interact with thiol containing enzymes that are involved in virus replication, thus hampering their functions. The cells when exposed to Ag^+ ions at similar concentration has been reported of not inhibiting the virus replication, due to which researchers concluded that antiviral property of Ag NCs (nanoclusters) was independent of the release of Ag(I) [48]. The mechanisms of Ag^+ ions and Ag NCs entrance into cells are reported to be different; therefore, their circulation and handling inside cells would be different. The difference so mentioned results into various forms of toxic actions for Ag ions and Ag NCs towards the viruses infecting the cells. For example, Ag NCs are reported to aggregate in the intracellular areas where important stages of the virus cycle are reported to be performed. Second, it has been reported that the antiviral competence of Ag NPs has been derived from the interaction of Ag NPs with the surface of viruses, which obstructs the docking on host cells thereby limiting their infectivity. Elechiguerra et al. have reported that the most favourable size of Ag NPs is around 10 nm, with somewhat larger or smaller NP sizes weaker physical interaction with the virus takes place. Orlowski et al. have reported that larger the NP, more efficiently it restricts the attachment of virus to host cell. It has been reported that docking of Ag NPs on virus surface has been related with the discharge of ROS from the surface destroying the virus membrane. Loaded Ag NPs on filters has reported to show efficient antiviral activity against bacteriophage MS2 [61].

Silver NPs Interaction with HCQ (CQ)

The active sites available in the compounds HCQ and CQ reports the charge distribution and their interaction with the noble metals like Ag and Au nanoparticles. The preliminary structure of the complex so formed by introducing a tiny cluster of Ag near the sites with abundant electrons has been reported. The electron rich sites are supposed to provide the electron density through their available lone pairs to 4*d* and 5*s* orbitals of Ag atom [62, 63]. In the compounds of CQ and HCQ, it has been reported that the Nitrogen present in the pyridine ring and the Oxygen of the hydroxyl group have got more attraction to interact with the clusters of noble metals. The optimized structure of HCQ and CQ on bilayer reports the attraction of the drug compounds for surface of Pt, the transfer and accumulation of charge on its surface have been confirmed via charge density difference. A stable icosahedral structure of Ag 147 and Au 147 NPs complexed with HCQ has been reported. It has been reported the non-covalent partially negative charge with viral receptors. Particle sizes of these NPs are groups which play important part in determining the potential of nanoparticle to catch HCQ (CQ). The binding energy of HCQ reported with Au NP is more favourable than AgNP. Electron affinity of Au is more in comparison to Ag [64], has been reported to enhance the interaction energy of Au atoms with the lone pairs of HCQ confirmed by the density difference and accumulation of negative charges on surface of Au. The adsorption energy of Pt is reported to be 40% more than surface of Au.

It has been reported that the adsorption property of these nanoparticles of noble metals and their coating with HCQ/CQ as a potential candidate for COVID-19. The charge transfer interaction with N- and O-group of drugs that are reported to increase by replacing the type of metal nanoparticles element (Pt NP > Au NP > Au Ag NP > Ag NP) have been studied. These noble nanoparticles with low toxicity and antiviral activity are efficient for using HCQ/CQ and decrease side effects.

Gold-Based Antiviral Nanoparticles

Au NPs are reported to show efficient antiviral applications [65]. The inhibition by Au NPs reported to include restricting the virus particles thereby restricting their attachment to the cell and controlling its spread. Au NPs of particle size 10 nm are reported to be prepared using plant extracts as reducing agents via chemical reduction method [66]. These Au NPs reported to lessen the viral infections. The effect of Au NPs on the virus was reported because of their interaction important in determining their antiviral properties. The cell survival rate was reported to be high about 60% when the Au NPs of size 14 nm applied in culture medium with cells having influenza viruses. Table 2 gives the comparison of various AuNPs based on their synthesis procedure and applications.

The multivalent effect makes the large Au NPs a stronger binding force with the molecules of protein on virus surface. It has been reported for sizes controlling many surfactants were used in the medium of synthesis and their size dependent antiviral activities and compared [71, 72]. The specificity of Au NPS was reported to be improved using DNA-Au NPs conjugated network [68]. They show antiviral activities against respiratory syncytial virus (RSV). The cell survival rate was reported to be about 99% when both DNA-Au NPs and RSV virus were cultured together. The layer formed by DNA-Au NPs restricts the viral infections. Au NPs with different morphological structure show different mechanisms for antiviral activities. Antiviral mechanisms were reported for (45 nm × 10 nm) used against RSV [69]. The survival rate of cells using Au nanorods were reported to be 82% in 2.5 μg/mL. The toxicity of Au has been reported to be reduced which enhances its abilities. Au NPs/LDHs are reported to show efficient antiviral properties at lower concentrations and the survival rate of cell after hepatitis B virus (HBV) infection was about 90% [70]. The Au released interacts with virus to trap them in cell and restrict their transmission. Due to their high cost, their utilizations are reported to be limited.

Table 2 Comparison of various types of Au NPs

S. No.	Types	Synthesis methods	Applications	References
1	Au NPs Particle size = 10 nm	Prepared using plant extracts as reducing agent	Lessens viral infections	[66]
2	Au NPs Particle size = 2 and 14 nm	Using sialic acid terminated glycerol dendrite as ligand	For 14 nm cell survival rate = 60% Effective against influenza virus	[67]
3	DNA-Au NPs	DNA-Au NPs conjugated network	Cell survival rate = 99% Effective against respiratory syncytial virus (RSV)	[68]
4	Au nanorods	–	Cell survival rate = 82% Effective against respiratory syncytial virus (RSV)	[69]
5	Au NPs/LDH	–	Cell survival rate = 90% Effective against Hepatitis B virus (HSV)	[70]

Inactivation of Virus Using Gold NPs

It has been reported Au NPs when capped with mercapto ethane sulfonate are efficient to inhibit HSV type 1 infection are potential to bind the virus. The NPs whose size has been reported to be equal or larger than virus are efficient in inhibiting the binding of virus to host cell, like polyvalent sulphated AuNPs [73]. Papp et al. reported Au NPs when coated with SA are efficient in inhibiting the binding of the influenza virus to that of target cells [67]. Cagno et al. have reported the antiviral NPs like Au and iron oxide core having these long and more flexible linker's effectively binding and inactivating viruses [20]. All these reported studies provide strong proof that these NPs are potent to be effective as antivirals.

Copper-Based Antiviral Nanoparticles

Few studies have been reported which states the antiviral properties of CuO NPs. It has been stated that the metal oxide has the potential of destructing the virus along with its genome. CuO NPs have been reported to show potential anti-HSV-1 virus efficiency when they are cultured together with the virus survival rate of cell reported to be 83.3% and non-toxic concentration 100 μg/mL [74].

The production of reactive oxygen species has been reported to be catalyzed by the release of Cu ions having the potential to disintegrate HSV degrading its genome. CuO NPs are reported to be applied in protective antiviral face mask [75]. The NPs has been reported to kill the virions in mask. Cu_2O NPs are also reported to be used for antiviral applications. Its antiviral potential has been studied against hepatitis C virus (HCV) [76]. HCV when treated with Cu_2O NPs infection rate reported to be reduced by 90%. Cu_2O NPs restricts the attachment and entry of HCV to host cells. Table 3 is the comparison of various CuNPs based on their applications.

Multiphase Cu_xO_y has been reported to be prepared by heating at various temperatures [78]. According to the zeta potential measurements, Cu_2O has been reported to have isoelectronic point of 11.0, and therefore, it is more effective to react with the viruses [79]. CuI nanoparticles of size 160 nm antiviral properties have also been reported [77]. They exhibit antiviral ability against HIN1influenza A virus. CuI has been reported to produce hydroxyl radicals which have potential to inactivate the virus. Cu_2S and CuCl have also been reported to be effective against infections [80].

2.2 *Metal Oxides as Antiviral Nanoparticles*

Various metal oxide NPs are reported to be having antiviral properties and are utilized as the antiviral agents. Figure 4 illustrates some of the metal oxide NPs with antiviral properties. The entry of HSV-1 into the target has been reported to be due

Table 3 Comparison of various types of Cu NPs

S. No.	Types	Applications	References
1	CuO NPs	Effective against HSV-1 Cell survival rate 83.3%	[74]
2	Cu_2O NPs	Effective against HCV [hepatitis C virus] Cell survival rate 98%	[76]
3	CuI	Effective against H1N1 influenza A virus	[77]

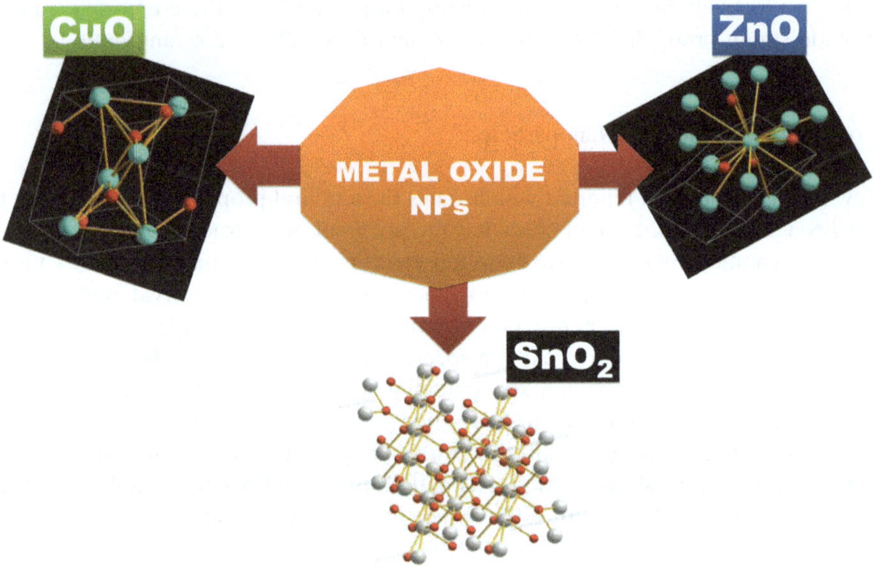

Fig. 4 The figure illustrates some of the metal oxide NPs with antiviral properties

to the interactions between glycoproteins which are wrapped by positive charged viral envelop and surface of the heparan sulphate which is negatively charged. The transmission into the cell has been designated as the first step which has been reported to be assisted by the introduction of HS-rich filopodia-like structures on the cell surface. The HSV-1 pathogenesis has been reported to be targeted using the ZnOMNSs (zinc oxide micro-nano structures) attached with nanoscopic spikes. The reported MNSs attack the virus to fight for its attachment to HS via their vacant oxygen sites present on the nanoscopic spikes affecting their infection and spread. According to the studies reported, the ZnO–MNSs which are partially negative are potential to capture the virions using the virostatic mechanism inactivating them to enter into the corneal fibroblasts. It has been reported that upon UV-light illumination extra vacancies of oxygen improving their ability against HSV-1. So the zinc oxide NP which is negatively charged has been reported to trap the herpes virus and restrict its interaction with the host cells [81]. The synthesized zinc oxide and silica nanoparticles are reported to be effective against Tobacco mosaic virus (TMV) infection in vitro and in vivo. According to the studies reported, TMV shows considerable aggregation and rupture in vitro after treatment with NPs. The cell survival rate reported to increase by 50% when ZnO was cultured with viruses. ZnO NPs inhibition ability on HSV-1 has been reported [82, 83]. TiO_2 NPs samples were reported to be prepared with tetragonal orientation and particle size of 8 nm via Sonochemical procedure [84]. It is reported to show good antiviral activity against new castle disease virus (NDV). Inhibition mechanism includes destroying the membrane of lipid and restricting the attachment of virus. Other metal oxides like SnO_2 nanowires are reported to be a potential inhibitor of entry to virus and its spread. SnO_2 concentrations used are reported to be below cytotoxic levels. A 75% reduction in the entry to cell has been reported with about 77% of clusters of infected cells and 99% of cell-to-cell fusion. These are reported to be effective anti-HSV agents and prophylactic agent [85]. The procedure of attaching gallium in glucan particles for its delivery into the immune cells has been reported in the studies. The evaluation for the anti-HIV infection properties of gallium has been studied. The GP-Ga_2 $(CO_3)_3$ reported to restrict inhibition of HIV growth up to 95% more than free Ga_2 $(CO_3)_3$ nanoparticles. They are reported to be potential delivery system for blocking the HIV infection of macrophages [86].

The researchers report developing iron oxide nanoparticles (IO-NPs) having a particle size of 10–15 nm which is effective to combat influenza strain A/H1N1/Eastern India/66/PR8-H1N1. They have studied its cell viability along with its anti-influenza properties and its restricting ability towards plaque. They report a cell feasibility of 50% at 4.25 pg $\pm$ 0.2 pg of iron oxide nanoparticles. As investigated, it has been reported about 08-fold reduction in the viral infection within 24 h when treated with iron oxide nanoparticles which is a new breakthrough for the use of IP-NPs against viral infections [87]. For the iron oxide NPs, its antiviral ability has been reported to be measured from the reduced ratio of the viral suspensions after the treatment. Because of its small size, it easily interacts with the virus and shows higher inhibition at low dosages. The interaction leads to restricting the virus from infecting the host cells [88].

As reported from the findings, the relationship between antiviral activity and the concentration of NPs implies the interaction between virion and composites. Molecular mechanism has been reported to be assumed a reaction between iron oxide and eSH group of proteins present in the cell leading to the inactivation of proteins [89]. Pure and single phase CeO_2 NPs ($\sim$14 nm) were reported to be synthesized from fruit extracts of *Hyphaene thebaica,* and its properties have been reported. These NPs are reported to have wide anti-microbial, antiviral as well as antioxidant properties. They are reported to be effective against poliovirus. Its potential against virus has been reported to be determined via cell feasibility of RD cells infected with the polio virus and its treatment with CeO_2 NPs [90].

CuO NPs have been reported to be synthesized using fruit extract of Syzygium alternifolium which shows antiviral properties against newcastle disease virus (NDV). It has been reported to show growth inhibitory effect on the virus [91]. Iron oxide NPs which are loaded on fibre glass has been reported to show antiviral activities against model virus, MS2 phage. It has been reported that the inactivation rate of Ag-modified Fe_2O_3 impregnated fibreglass (FG-Fe_2O_3/Ag) system was comparable to previously reported Ag nanoparticle impregnated fibreglass [92].

A docking study has been reported exploring the interaction of IONPs (Fe_2O_3 and Fe_3O_4) with the spike protein receptor required by virus for infecting the host cells. The analysis was reported to be done with hepatitis C virus (HCV) glycoproteins E1 and E2. According to the observation reported both Fe_2O_3 and Fe_3O_4 found efficient with the SARS-CoV-2 S1-RBD and to HCV glycoproteins, E1 and E2. Fe_3O_4 have been reported to form a more stable complex with S1-RBD and Fe_2O_3 favoured HCV E1 and E2. The interaction of IONPs has been expected to inactivate virus [93].

2.3 Photo Sensitizers as Antiviral Candidates

Photo sensitizers are reported as hydrophobic and in aqueous medium are reported to which affects their photochemical and photo biological characteristics [94, 95]. Figure 5 shows some of the photosensitising materials. Lim et al. reported a possible mechanism using NPs for photodynamic inactivation of viruses, preparation of $NaYF_4$ up conversion NPs (UCNs) along with zinc phthalocyanine photo sensitizers on their surface. The UCNs are reported to be coated with polyethylenimine making them hydrophilic and more flexible to manipulate. The UCNs are reported to show antiviral properties against dengue virus stereotype 2 and adenovirus type 5 [96]. MXenes [97, 98] are reported to be 2D transition metals of carbides, nitrides and carbon nitrides [99, 100] showing absorption maxima in the IR range and promising performance in the photodynamic and theranostic applications [101].

The carbon allotropes like fullerene and graphene are also reported to be potential candidates for inactivating virus via PDT [102]. So, exploring such types of nanomaterials based on photodynamic protocols could be helpful to inactivate SARS-CoV-2.

2.4 Halogen, Oxygen and Nitrogen Species as Potential Antiviral Candidates

Various important biological species like reactive Halogens, Nitrogen and Oxygen species have been reported to be vital and play physiological roles in living beings from plants to humans. It has been reported to include the superoxide dismutases (SOD); the catalytic enzymes for the formation of H_2O_2 which are necessary for protection of ROS induced injury in cell metabolism. The amount of ROS/RNS obtained by the ionizing radiation clinically at applicable doses has been reported to

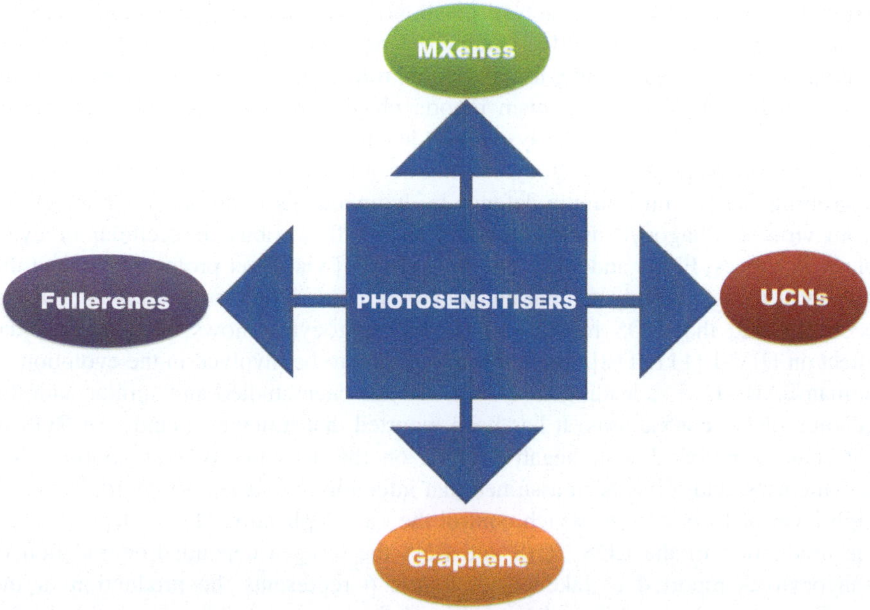

Fig. 5 This figure illustrates some of the photosensitizing materials

be ~1000 folds lesser than endogenous ROS/RNS level normally produced in a cell and RHS is reported to be vital in phagocytosis for immune defence. They have reported a reasonable strengthening mechanism for immune defence. It has been reported that H_2O_2 acts as a protective signalling molecule for the defence system in our body and its dysfunction leads to diseases like autoimmune disorders, ageing and cancer. A series of potential drug candidates are reported to be identified for treating pathogens like HIV and SARS-CoV-2 (COVID-19), cancer with mechanism of the drug activity. MOA of drugs have been reported, drug candidates like FMDs increases and does not restrict the endogenous pathogen killing effect present in human immune system. The halogenated aromatic drugs are reported to be utilized for experimental treatment of COVID-19. According to studies, there has been a constant production of the species like superoxide ($O_2^{\cdot-}$), (H_2O_2) and ($OH^{\cdot-}$) in aerobic metabolism of cell where hydroxyl radical is reported to be efficient, but non-selective oxidant, superoxide and hydrogen peroxide are less reactive in comparison. As per studies peroxide has been reported to be an important signalling molecule in various biological processes [103–107]. Peroxide is also reported to be signalling molecule of plant's defence mechanism against the pathogens [108]. The studies so reported states the vital role of superoxide dismutases (SOD) in humans and mammals, and these are the enzymes reported to convert superoxide to hydrogen peroxide [109]. The fast release of reactive species from cells like myeloid cells is reported as respiratory burst mostly used for immunological defence mechanisms. It has been stated that engulfed pathogens are destroyed when exposed to ROS (reactive oxygen species), RHS (reactive halogen species) or RNS (reactive nitrogen species) [110]. The process reported to be used by cell to engulf a pathogen forming phagosome. It plays a vital role in the immune defence efficiently killing pathogens. The mechanism reports phagosome moving to centrosome of phagocyte and fusing with the lysosomes leading to formation of phagolysosome degrading the pathogens. Phagocytosis has been mentioned to be efficient in killing microorganisms, with immune defence by lymphocytes importantly for infections from viruses. Phagocytosis is important as it kills various intracellular or cytoplasmic viruses, Ebola and HIV [56, 96, 111–114] via direct protection against the viruses or using antibody cellular phagocytosis for virus clearance [115–117]. It has been reported that ROS regulated RHS by phagocytes shows effective viricidal effect on HIV-1 [111, 112]. The bats are reported to be involved in the evolution of human SARS-CoV-2 leading to COVID-19 has been studied and similar with the genome of bat coronavirus. It has been reported that a higher quantity of ROS in bats has been found with negative effect on the activities of coronavirus RNA polymerases, and it has been assumed that infection in bats is asymptomatic due to high level of ROS present which control the viral replication [118]. Depending on the production of the ROS, RHS and RNS the oxygen depended degradation in phagocytosis reported to take place. Figure 6 represents the production of the reactive species utilized in pathogen degradation.

Firstly, it has been reported that NADPH oxidase which is embedded in the phagolysosome membrane activates to form $O_2^{\cdot-}$ by O_2 captivating an electron from the cytosolic NADPH. H_2O_2 has been reported to be obtained from $O_2^{\cdot-}$ using superoxide dismutases (SOD) or haem peroxides (MPO, EPO and LPO). The species $OH^{\cdot}$ have been reported to be generated through Haber—Weiss reaction. H_2O_2 has been reported to activate the halogen system via haem peroxides generating hypochlorous acid (HOCl) which helps in killing the pathogens [119–124]. All the ROS, RHS and RNS are reported to be strong oxidants capable of degrading the DNA/RNA, lipids, proteins and have got anti-pathogen effects [119–126]. HOCl has been reported to be used as disinfectant, whereas HOBr and HOI are identified in stimulated immune cells at lower levels [119–123]. Since, the macrophages are reported to have weaker antiviral properties than those of neutrophils. So, using respiratory burst these are activated which regulates inflammatory responses by synthesis of cytokines for redox signalling. When people affected by SARS-CoV-2 start to show symptoms and do not receive the treatments timely then they reported to develop symptoms of severe respiratory burst. In the case of respiratory burst, the halogen cyclic killing reactions reports to lead to disorders of related cell organelles and destroys the host cells and tissues. Due to enhanced RHS reactions, the excess toxicity caused leads to mutations of cell components and also affects signal pathway of H_2O_2 and $NO^{\cdot}$. The damages in the cell organelles affect organs and even lead to fatality. The treatment must be in preliminary stage.

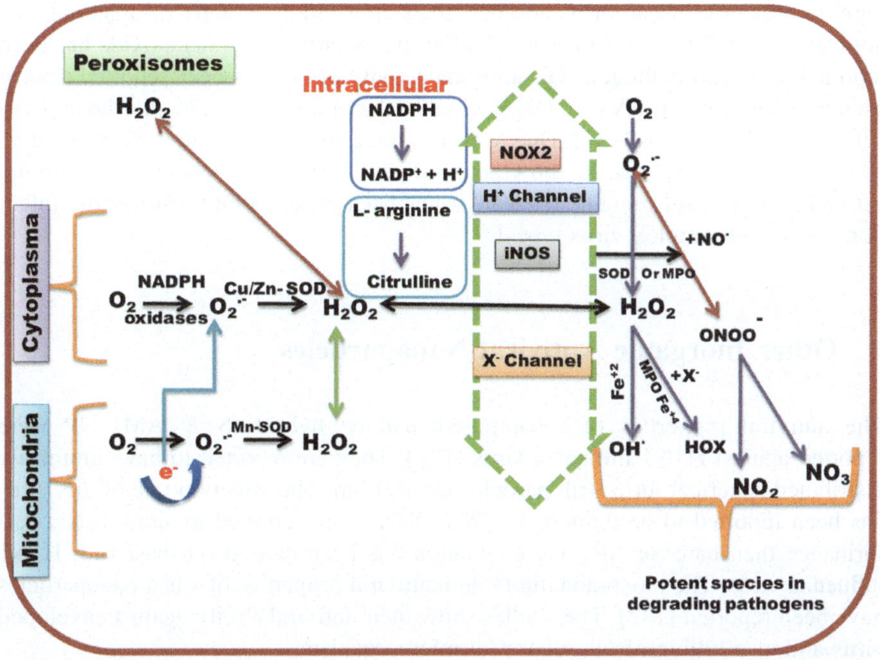

Fig. 6 This figure illustrates the production of reactive species for pathogen degradation, adapted and modified from Ref. [133]

3 Non-Metal Nanomaterials as Antiviral Materials

3.1 Carbon-Based Antiviral Materials

The atoms of carbon are reported to link with each other in various ways amongst each other resulting in different allotropes like carbon dots, carbon nanotubes and graphene oxide. These carbon allotropes have been reported to be studied in terms of their anti-microbial properties along with their physical and chemical properties. The anti-infection potential of these carbon compounds has been reported because of their geometry. Investigations regarding the antiviral activity of these compounds have also been reported. The effect of carbon dots on pseudorabies virus (PRV) also on porcine reproductive and respiratory syndrome virus (PRRSV) [127]. When the infected cells are treated with carbon dots, it has been reported the infection was reduced to 80%. It has been reported that carbon dots restrict the multiplication of the PRV and PRRSV. The surface properties of the carbon dots are reported to be the factor affecting its safety and biocompatibility. There has been reports of preparation of a core shell carbon dot sample via dry heat treatment of curcumin and its antiviral activity has been studied against enterovirus 71 (EV71) [128]. The inhibition rate against the infection of virus was reported to exceed 99%. Due to high cytotoxicity of carbon nanotubes, their application as antiviral materials are not clear [129]. The two-dimensional allotrope of carbon, graphene oxide has been reported to be anti-pathogen. The antiviral activity of GO has been reported against pseudorabies virus [PRV], a DNA virus and porcine epidemic diarrhoea virus [PEDV], an RNA virus [130]. Due to their unique single layer and surface negative charges, they are reported to show antiviral activities. The mechanism of antiviral activities of GO still remains unclear. It has been reported GO restricts the infections of herpes simplex virus type-1.

4 Other Inorganic Antiviral Nanoparticles

The antiviral properties of selenium-adamantine hybrid (Se@ AM) NP were reported against H1N1 influenza virus [131]. They are reported to have uniformly distributed spherical form with particle size 100 nm. The infection rate of this virus has been reported to be reduced by 79%. SeNPs are reported to show better performance than bare Se NPs and evaluation has been carried out based on H1N1 influenza virus. The biocompatibility and antiviral properties of silica nanoparticles have been reported [132]. The studies show their antiviral ability against enveloped virus and also killing of other harmful microorganisms.

5 Conclusion

COVID-19 outbreak has reportedly been declared as a global pandemic and people worldwide are facing many unparalleled challenges. The current situation needs communal thinking which would be helpful for unified and inter-reliant actions. The challenge can be addressed with the cooperation of the researchers worldwide with their expertise. It is an incredible prospect in terms of scientific contexts, methods involving various disciplines leading to exchange of knowledge increasing diversity to achieve the solutions. Till date, there are no competent antiviral drugs or vaccines available for treating COVID-19. The optimistic result is all the possible areas are explored counting antiviral drugs that are exists for other viral diseases are subjected to clinical assessment.

References

1. Amanat F, Krammer F (2020) SARS-CoV-2 vaccines: status report. Immunity 52(4):583–589
2. Chen WH et al (2020) The SARS-CoV-2 vaccine pipeline: an overview. Curr Trop Med Rep 1–4

3. Yadavalli T, Shukla D (2017) Role of metal and metal oxide nanoparticles as diagnostic and therapeutic tools for highly prevalent viral infections. Nanomedicine 13(1):219–230
4. Singh L et al (2017) The role of nanotechnology in the treatment of viral infections. Ther Adv Infect Dis 4(4):105–131
5. Jackman JA, Lee J, Cho NJ (2016) Nanomedicine for infectious disease applications: innovation towards broad-spectrum treatment of viral infections. Small 12(9):1133–1139
6. Adesina SK, Akala EO (2015) Nanotechnology approaches for the delivery of exogenous siRNA for HIV therapy. Mol Pharm 12(12):4175–4187
7. Mammen M, Choi S-K, Whitesides GM (1998) Polyvalent interactions in biological systems: implications for design and use of multivalent ligands and inhibitors. Angew Chem Int Ed 37(20):2754–2794
8. Fasting C et al (2012) Multivalency as a chemical organization and action principle. Angew Chem Int Ed Engl 51(42):10472–10498
9. Choppin PW, Scheid A (1980) The role of viral glycoproteins in adsorption, penetration, and pathogenicity of viruses. Rev Infect Dis 2(1):40–61
10. Sarrazin S, Lamanna WC, Esko JD (2011) Heparan sulfate proteoglycans. Cold Spring Harb Perspect Biol 3(7):a004952
11. Stencel-Baerenwald JE et al (2014) The sweet spot: defining virus-sialic acid interactions. Nat Rev Microbiol 12(11):739–749
12. Papp I et al (2011) Inhibition of influenza virus activity by multivalent glycoarchitectures with matched sizes. ChemBioChem 12(6):887–895
13. Bhatia S, Camacho LC, Haag R (2016) Pathogen inhibition by multivalent ligand architectures. J Am Chem Soc 138(28):8654–8666
14. Rusnati M et al (2009) Sulfated K5 Escherichia coli polysaccharide derivatives: a novel class of candidate antiviral microbicides. Pharmacol Ther 123(3):310–322
15. Tang S et al (2016) Antiviral agents from multivalent presentation of sialyl oligosaccharides on brush polymers. ACS Macro Lett 5(3):413–418
16. Dey P et al (2018) Multivalent flexible nanogels exhibit broad-spectrum antiviral activity by blocking virus entry. ACS Nano 12(7):6429–6442
17. Baram-Pinto D et al (2009) Inhibition of herpes simplex virus type 1 infection by silver nanoparticles capped with mercaptoethane sulfonate. Bioconjug Chem 20(8):1497–1502
18. Cheng HW et al (2018) Synthesis of S-linked NeuAc-α(2–6)-di-LacNAc bearing liposomes for H1N1 influenza virus inhibition assays. Bioorg Med Chem 26(9):2262–2270
19. van Dongen MJP et al (2019) A small-molecule fusion inhibitor of influenza virus is orally active in mice. Science 363(6431)
20. Cagno V et al (2018) Broad-spectrum non-toxic antiviral nanoparticles with a virucidal inhibition mechanism. Nat Mater 17(2):195–203
21. Zhou P et al (2020) A pneumonia outbreak associated with a new coronavirus of probable bat origin. Nature 579(7798):270–273
22. Monteil V et al (2020) Inhibition of SARS-CoV-2 infections in engineered human tissues using clinical-grade soluble human ACE2. Cell 181(4):905-913.e7
23. Zhang H et al (2020) Angiotensin-converting enzyme 2 (ACE2) as a SARS-CoV-2 receptor: molecular mechanisms and potential therapeutic target. Intensive Care Med 46(4):586–590
24. Hoffmann M et al (2020) SARS-CoV-2 cell entry depends on ACE2 and TMPRSS2 and Is blocked by a clinically proven protease inhibitor. Cell 181(2):271-280.e8
25. Jones ST et al., *Modified cyclodextrins as broad-spectrum antivirals.* Science Advances, 2020. **6**(5): p. eaax9318.
26. Lukashev AN, Zamyatnin AA Jr (2016) Viral vectors for gene therapy: current state and clinical perspectives. Biochemistry (Mosc) 81(7):700–708
27. Anderson WF, Blaese RM, Culver K (1990) The ADA human gene therapy clinical protocol: points to consider response with clinical protocol. Hum Gene Ther 1(3):331–362
28. Walther W, Stein U (2000) Viral vectors for gene transfer. Drugs 60(2):249–271
29. Kostarelos K (2020) Nanoscale nights of COVID-19. Nat Nanotechnol 15:343
30. Yin H et al (2014) Non-viral vectors for gene-based therapy. Nat Rev Genet 15(8):541–555

31. Vincent M, de Lázaro I, Kostarelos K (2017) Graphene materials as 2D non-viral gene transfer vector platforms. Gene Ther 24(3):123–132
32. Lozano R et al (2012) Global and regional mortality from 235 causes of death for 20 age groups in 1990 and 2010: a systematic analysis for the Global Burden of Disease Study 2010. Lancet 380(9859):2095–2128
33. Watkins K (2018) Emerging infectious diseases: a review. Curr Emerg Hosp Med Rep 6:86–93
34. Rai M et al (2016) Strategic role of selected noble metal nanoparticles in medicine. Crit Rev Microbiol 42(5):696–719
35. Jeyaraj M, Gurunathan S, Qasim M, Kang M-H, Kim J-H (2019) A comprehensive review on the synthesis, characterization, and biomedical application of platinumnanoparticles. Nanomaterials 9:1719
36. Ravindra S et al (2012) Development and characterization of curcumin loaded silver nanoparticle hydrogels for antibacterial and drug delivery applications. J Inorg Organomet Polym Mater 22(6):1254–1262
37. Burduel A-C, Gherasim O, Grumezescu AM, Mogoant L, Ficai A, Andronescu E (2018) Biomedical applications of silver nanoparticles: an up-to-date overview. Nanomaterials 8 (681)
38. Peña Gonzalez CE, García Broncano P, Ottaviani MF, Cangiotti M, Fattori A, Hierro-Oliva M, Gonzalez-Martin ML, Perez-Serrano J, Gómez R, Muñoz Fernandez MA (2016) Dendronized anionic gold nanoparticles: synthesis, characterization, and antiviral activity. Chem—Euro J 22:2987–2999
39. Henke P, Kirakci K, Kubt P, Fraiberk M, Forstov J, Mosinger J (2016) Antibacterial, antiviral, and oxygen-sensing nanoparticles prepared from electrospun materials. ACS Appl Mater Interfaces 8:25127–25136
40. Galdiero S et al (2011) Silver nanoparticles as potential antiviral agents. Molecules 16 (10):8894–8918
41. Villeret B et al (2018) Silver nanoparticles impair retinoic acid-inducible gene I-mediated mitochondrial antiviral immunity by blocking the autophagic flux in lung epithelial cells. ACS Nano 12(2):1188–1202
42. Morris D et al (2019) Antiviral and immunomodulatory activity of silver nanoparticles in experimental RSV infection. Viruses 11(8)
43. Orlowski P, Kowalczyk A, Tomaszewska E, Ranoszek-Soliwoda K, Wegrzyn A, Grzesiak J, Celichowski G, Grobelny J, Eriksson K, Krzyzowska M (2018) Antiviral activity of tannic acid modified silver nanoparticles: potential to activate immune response in herpes genitalis. Viruses-Basel 10(524)
44. Huy TQ, Thanh NTH, Thy NT, Van Chung P, Hung PN, Le A-T, Hanh NTH (2017) Cytotoxicity and antiviral activity of electrochemical-synthesized silver nanoparticles against poliovirus. J Virol Methods 241:52
45. Lara H, Ayala-Nuñez NV, Turrent L-I, Rodriguez-Padilla C (2010) Mode of antiviral action of silver nanoparticles against HIV-1. J Nanobiotechnol 8(1)
46. Sharma V, Kaushik S, Pandit P, Dhull D, Yadav J, Kaushik S (2019) Green synthesis of silver nanoparticles from medicinal plants and evaluation of their antiviral potential against chikungunya virus. Appl Microbiol Biotechnol 103(881)
47. Li Y, Lin Z, Zhao M, Xu T, Wang C, Hua L, Wang H, Xia H, Zhu B (2016) Silver nanoparticle based codelivery of oseltamivir to inhibit the activity of the H1N1 influenza virus through ROS-mediated signaling pathways. ACS Appl Mater Interfaces 8:24385
48. Du T et al (2018) Glutathione-capped Ag2S nanoclusters inhibit coronavirus proliferation through blockage of viral RNA synthesis and budding. ACS Appl Mater Interfaces 10 (5):4369–4378
49. Li Y, Lin Z, Zhao M, Guo M, Xu T, Wang C, Xia H, Zhu B (2016) Reversal of H1N1 influenza virus-induced apoptosis by silver nanoparticles functionalized with amantadine. RSC Adv 6:89679

50. Lin Z, Li Y, Guo M, Xu T, Wang C, Zhao M, Wang H, Chen T, Zhu B (2017) The inhibition of H1N1 influenza virus-induced apoptosis by silver nanoparticles functionalized with zanamivir. RSC Adv 7:7420
51. Santos Pereira A, Nakahata D, Manzano C, Alencar Simoni D, Pereira D, Lustri W, Formiga A, Corbi P (2019) Synthesis, crystallographic studies, molecular modeling and in vitro biological studies of silver(I) complexes with aminoadamantane ligands. Polyhedron 173:114
52. Du T, Liang J, Dong N, Lu J, Fu Y, Fang L, Xiao S, Han H (2018) Glutathione-Capped Ag_2S nanoclusters inhibit coronavirus proliferation through blockage of viral RNA synthesis and budding. ACS Appl Mater Interfaces 10:4369
53. Seifullina I, Martsinko E, Gridina T, Chebanenko E, Mudrik L, Fedchuk A (2019) Antiviral properties of the new coordination compound silver bis(citrato)germanate. Pharm Chem J 53:318
54. Plotnikov E, Silnikov V, Gapeyev A, Plotnikov V (2016) Investigation of DNA-damage and chromosomal aberrations in blood cells under the influence of new silver-based antiviral complex. Adv Pharm Bull 6:71
55. Cavicchioli M, Massabni A, Heinrich T, Costa-Neto C, Abrao E, Fonseca B, Castellano E, Corbi P, Lustri W, Leite C (2010) Pt(II) and Ag(I) complexes with acesulfame: crystal structure and a study of their antitumoral, antimicrobial and antiviral activities. J Inorg Biochem 104:533
56. Rogers JV, Parkinson CV, Choi YW, Speshock JL, Hussain SM (2008) A preliminary assessment of silver nanoparticle inhibition of monkeypox virus plaque formation. Nanoscale Res Lett 3:129–133
57. De Gusseme B, Sintubin L, Baert L, Thibo E, Hennebel T, Vermeulen G, Uyttendaele M, Verstraete W, Boon N (2010) Biogenic silver for disinfection of water contaminated with viruses. Appl Environ Microbiol 76:1082–1087
58. Park S et al (2018) Disinfection of waterborne viruses using silver nanoparticle-decorated silica hybrid composites in water environments. Sci Total Environ 625:477–485
59. Orlowski P et al (2014) Tannic acid modified silver nanoparticles show antiviral activity in herpes simplex virus type 2 infection. PLoS One 9(8):e104113
60. Lu L et al (2008) Silver nanoparticles inhibit hepatitis B virus replication. Antivir Ther 13 (2):253–262
61. Joe YH, Park DH, Hwang J (2016) Evaluation of Ag nanoparticle coated air filter against aerosolized virus: anti-viral efficiency with dust loading. J Hazard Mater 301:547–553
62. Pakiari AH, Jamshidi Z (2007) Interaction of amino acids with gold and silver clusters. J Phys Chem A 111(20):4391–4396
63. Aliakbar Tehrani Z et al (2012) Interactions of glutathione tripeptide with gold cluster: influence of intramolecular hydrogen bond on complexation behavior. J Phys Chem A 116 (17):4338–4347
64. Granatier J, Urban M, Sadlej AJ (2007) Van der Waals complexes of Cu, Ag, and Au with hydrogen sulfide. The bonding character. J Phys Chem A 111(50):13238–13244
65. Lévy R et al (2004) Rational and combinatorial design of peptide capping ligands for gold nanoparticles. J Am Chem Soc 126(32):10076–10084
66. Meléndez-Villanueva MA et al (2019) Virucidal activity of gold nanoparticles synthesized by green chemistry using garlic extract. Viruses 11(12):1111
67. Papp I et al (2010) Inhibition of influenza virus infection by multivalent sialic-acid-functionalized gold nanoparticles. Small 6(24):2900–2906
68. Li CM et al (2016) DNA-AuNP networks on cell membranes as a protective barrier to inhibit viral attachment, entry and budding. Biomaterials 77:216–226
69. Bawage SS et al (2016) Gold nanorods inhibit respiratory syncytial virus by stimulating the innate immune response. Nanomed Nanotechnol Biol Med 12(8):2299–2310
70. Carja G et al (2015) Self-assemblies of plasmonic gold/layered double hydroxides with highly efficient antiviral effect against the hepatitis B virus. Nano Res 8(11):3512–3523

71. Tao W et al (2017) Consensus M2e peptide conjugated to gold nanoparticles confers protection against H1N1, H3N2 and H5N1 influenza A viruses. Antiviral Res 141:62–72
72. Chakravarthy KV et al (2010) Gold nanorod delivery of an ssRNA immune activator inhibits pandemic H1N1 influenza viral replication. Proc Natl Acad Sci USA 107(22):10172–10177
73. Vonnemann J et al (2014) Virus inhibition induced by polyvalent nanoparticles of different sizes. Nanoscale 6(4):2353–2360
74. Tavakoli A, Hashemzadeh MS (2020) Inhibition of herpes simplex virus type 1 by copper oxide nanoparticles. J Virol Methods 275:113688
75. Borkow G et al (2010) A novel anti-influenza copper oxide containing respiratory face mask. PLoS One 5(6):e11295
76. Hang X et al (2015) Antiviral activity of cuprous oxide nanoparticles against Hepatitis C Virus in vitro. J Virol Methods 222:150–157
77. Fujimori Y et al (2012) Novel antiviral characteristics of nanosized copper(I) iodide particles showing inactivation activity against 2009 pandemic H1N1 influenza virus. Appl Environ Microbiol 78(4):951–955
78. Mazurkow JM et al (2020) Nano-sized copper (oxide) on alumina granules for water filtration: effect of copper oxidation state on virus removal performance. Environ Sci Technol 54(2):1214–1222
79. Minoshima M et al (2016) Comparison of the antiviral effect of solid-state copper and silver compounds. J Hazard Mater 312:1–7
80. Sunada K, Minoshima M, Hashimoto K (2012) Highly efficient antiviral and antibacterial activities of solid-state cuprous compounds. J Hazard Mater 235–236:265–270
81. Mishra YK et al (2011) Virostatic potential of micro-nano filopodia-like ZnO structures against herpes simplex virus-1. Antiviral Res 92(2):305–312
82. Cai L et al (2019) Preventing viral disease by ZnONPs through directly deactivating TMV and activating plant immunity in Nicotiana benthamiana. Environ Sci Nano 6(12):3653–3669
83. Tavakoli A et al (2018) Polyethylene glycol-coated zinc oxide nanoparticle: an efficient nanoweapon to fight against herpes simplex virus type 1. Nanomedicine (Lond) 13(21): 2675–2690
84. Akhtar S et al (2019) Antibacterial and antiviral potential of colloidal Titanium dioxide (TiO_2) nanoparticles suitable for biological applications. Mater Res Express 6(10):105409
85. Trigilio J et al (2012) Tin oxide nanowires suppress herpes simplex virus-1 entry and cell-to-cell membrane fusion. PLoS One 7(10):e48147
86. Soto ER et al (2016) Targeted delivery of glucan particle encapsulated gallium nanoparticles inhibits HIV growth in human macrophages. J Drug Deliv 2016:8520629
87. Kumar R et al (2019) Iron oxide nanoparticles based antiviral activity of H1N1 influenza A virus. J Infect Chemother 25(5):325–329
88. Elechiguerra JL et al (2005) Interaction of silver nanoparticles with HIV-1. J Nanobiotechnology 3:6
89. Mori Y et al (2013) Antiviral activity of silver nanoparticle/chitosan composites against H1N1 influenza A virus. Nanoscale Res Lett 8(1):93–93
90. Mohamed HEA et al (2020) Promising antiviral, antimicrobial and therapeutic properties of green nanoceria. Nanomedicine (Lond) 15(5):467–488
91. Yugandhar P et al (2018) Cost effective, green synthesis of copper oxide nanoparticles using fruit extract of Syzygium alternifolium (Wt.) Walp., characterization and evaluation of antiviral activity. J Clust Sci 29(4):743–755
92. Nangmenyi G et al (2011) Silver-modified iron oxide nanoparticle impregnated fiberglass for disinfection of bacteria and viruses in water. Mater Lett 65:1191–1193
93. Abo-zeid Y et al (2020) A molecular docking study repurposes FDA approved iron oxide nanoparticles to treat and control COVID-19 infection. Eur J Pharm Sci 153:105465
94. Wainwright M (2003) Local treatment of viral disease using photodynamic therapy. Int J Antimicrob Agents 21(6):510–520

95. Lim ME et al (2012) Photodynamic inactivation of viruses using upconversion nanoparticles. Biomaterials 33(6):1912–1920
96. Peterhans E et al (1987) Virus-induced formation of reactive oxygen intermediates in phagocytic cells. Free Radical Res Commun 3(1–5):39–46
97. Naguib M et al (2011) Two-dimensional nanocrystals produced by exfoliation of Ti_3AlC_2. Adv Mater 23(37):4248–4253
98. Naguib M et al (2011) Synthesis of a new nanocrystalline titanium aluminum fluoride phase by reaction of Ti_2AlC with hydrofluoric acid. RSC Adv 1(8):1493–1499
99. Urbankowski P et al (2016) Synthesis of two-dimensional titanium nitride Ti_4N_3 (MXene). Nanoscale 8(22):11385–11391
100. Naguib M et al (2012) Two-dimensional transition metal carbides. ACS Nano 6(2):1322–1331
101. Anasori B, Gogotsi Y (2019) Introduction to 2D transition metal carbides and nitrides (MXenes). In: Anasori B, Gogotsi Y (eds) 2D metal carbides and nitrides (MXenes): structure, properties and applications. Springer International Publishing, Cham, pp 3–12
102. Wiehe A, O'Brien JM, Senge MO (2019) Trends and targets in antiviral phototherapy. Photochem Photobiol Sci 18(11):2565–2612
103. Rhee SG (2006) Cell signaling. H_2O_2, a necessary evil for cell signaling. Science 312(5782): 1882–1883
104. Veal EA, Day AM, Morgan BA (2007) Hydrogen peroxide sensing and signaling. Mol Cell 26(1):1–14
105. Watson JD (2014) Type 2 diabetes as a redox disease. Lancet 383(9919):841–843
106. Lambeth JD, Neish AS (2014) Nox enzymes and new thinking on reactive oxygen: a double-edged sword revisited. Annu Rev Pathol 9:119–145
107. Sies H (2017) Hydrogen peroxide as a central redox signaling molecule in physiological oxidative stress: oxidative eustress. Redox Biol 11:613–619
108. Torres MA, Jones JDG, Dangl JL (2006) Reactive oxygen species signaling in response to pathogens. Plant Physiol 141(2):373–378
109. McCord JM, Fridovich I (1969) Superoxide dismutase. An enzymic function for erythrocuprein (hemocuprein). J Biol Chem 244(22):6049–55
110. Lehnert S (2007) Biomolecular action of ionizing radiation, 1st edn. CRC Press
111. Chase MJ, Klebanoff SJ (1992) Viricidal effect of stimulated human mononuclear phagocytes on human immunodeficiency virus type 1. Proc Natl Acad Sci USA 89(12): 5582–5585
112. Klebanoff SJ, Coombs RW (1992) Viricidal effect of polymorphonuclear leukocytes on human immunodeficiency virus-1. Role of the myeloperoxidase system. J Clin Invest 89 (6):2014–2017
113. Kramer M et al (2008) Phagocytosis of picornavirus-infected cells induces an RNA-dependent antiviral state in human dendritic cells. J Virol 82(6):2930–2937
114. Vangeti S, Yu M, Smed-Sörensen A (2018) Respiratory mononuclear phagocytes in human influenza A virus infection: their role in immune protection and as targets of the virus. Front Immunol 9:1521–1521
115. Van Strijp JA et al (1989) Complement-mediated phagocytosis of herpes simplex virus by granulocytes. Binding or ingestion. J Clin Invest 84(1):107–112
116. Powell RLR et al (2019) Primary human neutrophils exhibit a unique HIV-directed antibody-dependent phagocytosis profile. J Innate Immun 11(2):181–190
117. Tay MZ, Wiehe K, Pollara J (2019) Antibody-dependent cellular phagocytosis in antiviral immune responses. Front Immunol 10:332
118. Zhang G et al (2013) Comparative analysis of bat genomes provides insight into the evolution of flight and immunity. Science 339(6118):456–460
119. Albrich JM, McCarthy CA, Hurst JK (1981) Biological reactivity of hypochlorous acid: implications for microbicidal mechanisms of leukocyte myeloperoxidase. Proc Natl Acad Sci USA 78(1):210–214

120. Arnhold J et al (2006) Kinetics and thermodynamics of halide and nitrite oxidation by mammalian heme peroxidases. Eur J Inorg Chem 2006(19):3801–3811
121. Davies MJ et al (2008) Mammalian heme peroxidases: from molecular mechanisms to health implications. Antioxid Redox Signal 10(7):1199–1234
122. Slauch JM (2011) How does the oxidative burst of macrophages kill bacteria? Still an open question. Mol Microbiol 80(3):580–583
123. Aratani Y (2018) Myeloperoxidase: its role for host defense, inflammation, and neutrophil function. Arch Biochem Biophys 640:47–52
124. Beckman JS et al (1990) Apparent hydroxyl radical production by peroxynitrite: implications for endothelial injury from nitric oxide and superoxide. Proc Natl Acad Sci USA 87(4):1620–1624
125. McCafferty DM (2000) Peroxynitrite and inflammatory bowel disease. Gut 46(3):436–439
126. Radi R (2018) Oxygen radicals, nitric oxide, and peroxynitrite: redox pathways in molecular medicine. Proc Natl Acad Sci 115(23):5839–5848
127. Du T et al (2016) Carbon dots as inhibitors of virus by activation of type I interferon response. Carbon 110:278–285
128. Lin C-J et al (2019) High amplification of the antiviral activity of curcumin through transformation into carbon quantum dots. Small 15(41):1902641
129. Chen H et al (2019) Single-walled carbon nanotubes repress viral-induced defense pathways through oxidative stress. Nanotoxicology 13(9):1176–1196
130. Ye S et al (2015) Antiviral activity of graphene oxide: how sharp edged structure and charge matter. ACS Appl Mater Interfaces 7(38):21571–21579
131. Li Y et al (2018) Inhibition of H1N1 influenza virus-induced apoptosis by functionalized selenium nanoparticles with amantadine through ROS-mediated AKT signaling pathways. Int J Nanomed 13:2005–2016
132. de Souza e Silva JM et al (2016) Viral inhibition mechanism mediated by surface-modified silica nanoparticles. ACS Appl Mater Interfaces 8(26):16564–16572
133. Bin Lu Q (2020) Reaction cycles of halogen species in the immune defense: implications for human health and diseases and the pathology and treatment of COVID-19. Cells 9(6). https://doi.org/10.3390/cells9061461

Chapter 5
Perspective of Organic-Based Antimicrobial Coating Materials: Implication Toward COVID-19

Benjamin Raj, Arun Kumar Padhy, Suddhasatwa Basu, and Mamata Mohapatra

1 Introduction

Recently incipient infectious ailments caused by virus has established the forefront of global health concerns. Nowadays the entire world is suffering the eruption of typical pneumonia caused by novel coronavirus SAR-CoV-2 (2019-nCoV). In December 2019 a novel coronavirus was reported in the Wuhan city of China including thousands of deaths led to a pandemic for the respiratory system. On March 11, 2020, the WHO declared the COVID-19 outbreak a pandemic [1]. Now it has been spread almost all over the world with millions of infections and lacs of death. It also devastated the economy and took a toll healthcare worldwide. From the report, it is concluded that the structure of this virus is spherical with some pleomorphism having diameter 60–140 nm and the surface covered with some of the spike like morphology with an average range of 9–13 nm [2]. The main symptoms of COVID-19 are fever, cough, headache, loss of appetite, sore throat, vomiting diarrhea, abdominal pain, and fatigue. The brutality of disease not only depends on the COVID-19 virus but also depends on the comorbidities such as high blood pressure, sugar (diabetes), kidney-related problems, and coronary heart disease, respectively [3]. The incubation period reported for the patients is in between 5 and 14 days before disease started. Recently, reported data indicate that patients who is suffering from COVID-19 also exhibits damages of kidney, liver, heart, and nervous system a brain (encephalitis). Almost entire world is now suffering from this pandemic. Till date there are few therapeutic and no vaccine has been invented to control this pandemic. The rapid diagnosis, tracking/surveillance, and case isolation/quarantine are some of the primarily preventive measures to stop the

B. Raj · S. Basu · M. Mohapatra
CSIR-Institute of Minerals and Materials Technology, Bhubaneswar, Odisha 751013, India

A. K. Padhy (✉)
Department of Chemistry, Central University of Jharkhand, Ranchi 835205, India
e-mail: arun.padhy@cuj.ac.in

M. Mohapatra et al. (eds.), *COVID-19 Pandemic*, Materials Horizons: From Nature to Nanomaterials, https://doi.org/10.1007/978-981-16-4372-9_5

spread of this novel coronavirus. These viruses transmit from one infected person to another by inhalation or emission of body fluid during the sneezing, or aerosol particle comprising virus which subsequently attached to the surface and gets attached with the receiver person. Aerosolized pathogens are the principal source for the respiratory infections and their body-to-body transmissions cycle. It also plays an important role in spreading of viruses in the air. There are several safety measures to control the communal transmission like sanitizing hand with sanitizer, washing hand regularly for at least 22 s, keeping social distancing of minimum 1 m in the enclosed or public places, hand gloves, and face mask. However, most of the face mask is not authenticated or enough to control the effect of coronaviruses spread. The antimicrobial textiles have attracted a great attention to the researcher with the goals of reducing the transmission of microbes from one person to another and improving the life quality of human beings. The airborne transmission intertwines system and respiratory protection against the novel coronaviruses and is presented in Fig. 1.

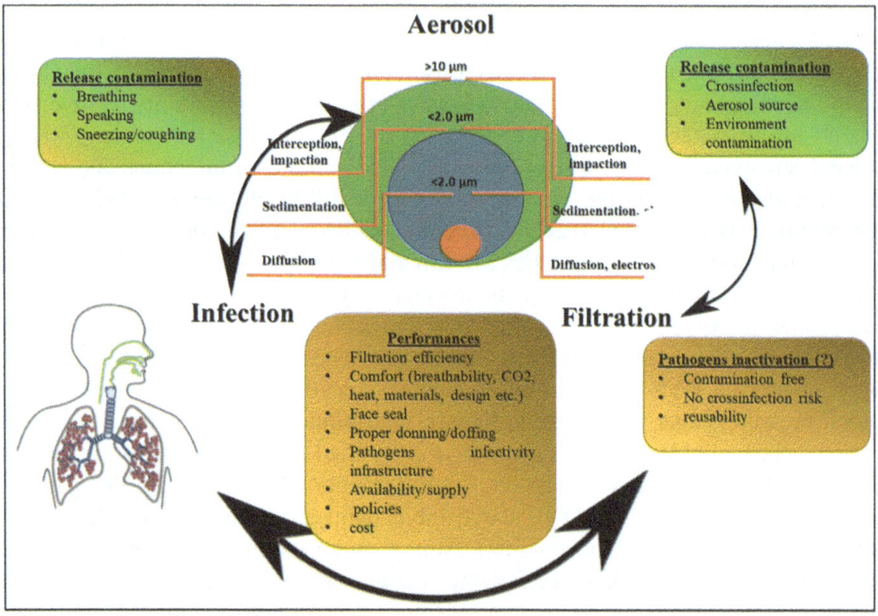

Fig. 1 Respiratory protection and airborne transmission intertwine system. Reproduced with permission [2]

In this chapter, we will discuss about mode of spreading, problems, and preventive measures to control the spread of coronaviruses. Meanwhile we also briefly reviewed the recent research progress toward the antiviral coating materials including organic precursors as antiviral coating agent on textile that have been used as face mask. Lastly, we also focussed on challenges and future perspectives of the applications of advanced organic material for antiviral coating agent.

2 Modes of Spreading of Virus

Various factors responsible for the spread of coronavirus are identified in the literature that affects and dominates air droplet transportation are listed as: size of the droplet, humidity, temperature, and human gathering/clustering. As per the reported data high temperature and humidity diminish the fortuitous of transmission of COVID-19 [4]. There is direct relation between the speed of airflow and the propagation of pathogenic aerosol droplets when the people breathe, talk, coughing and sneezing, etc. The dispersion of aerosol at molecular level depends upon various mechanical and air-surface that provide energy for bond breaking between droplet and host cellular surface. The kinetics of transmission of viruses depends upon the size of droplets and speed respectively. The higher the speed, longer the distances and the longer travel time. If the size of the droplet will be bigger it will easily settle down whereas if size of droplet will be small it will evaporate faster than they settle. The infectious disease can also spread through many other ways such as person-to-person spread (needle injection, cloth, furniture, utensils (fomites), sexual transmission, etc.), common vehicles, food-borne, water-borne blood products, etc. The most common transmission of the viruses occurs through the fomites which are responsible for spreading and also acts as reservoirs for the growth of microbes [5]. When the person come in contact with infected person, these notorious viruses can easily transferred to healthy one. The pathogenic microbes were deposited over the surface of day-to-day life objects like doors, knobs, calling bell, telephones, and toys, when an infected person touched all above leading to the perpetual spreading of infections. The various human activities like coughing in public places, sneezing, breathing, even talking which produces aerosolized moisture droplets containing bacteria. Anyone who is within 6 ft. of that infected person can have breathed it and gets contamination. The coronavirus exists in the air upon 3 h which can easily be transferred to the lungs of healthy person.

The coronaviruses most oftenly transmitted/spread through a person who has some symptoms as shown in Fig. 2. Some time people who don't know they have infected from novel coronaviruses can also bear a carrier for the transmission of this deadly diseases which is called asymptomatic spread. From the report, it is expected that asymptomatic types of spread are dangerous and are a major drivers for the growth of COVID-19 pandemic [6]. And a person who is transmitting these viruses before any symptoms is called presymptomatic spread. Whereas some people can trace how they can get the virus because they know that they have been in contact with someone who is sick called community spread.

3 Challenges to Control the Transmission of COVID-19

A number of challenges have been considered to prevent the spread of COVID-19. The lack of medical appliances supplies (shortages of mask, safety goggles) and advanced laboratory facilities to test for effectively and widely. One of the major challenges for the doctors and scientific community is to identify the asymptomatic patients having no any symptoms. As it transmits from one person to another with direct contact, therefore, it is the major challenge to avoid the public gathering, unnecessary movement, departures of busses and trains. The whole world is now facing the shortage of medical equipment, medicine, vaccine, and economical crisis as well, especially the availability of N-95 mask. Therefore, it is prime necessities to develop the effective devices (masks, PPE kit, and hand gloves) or medical appliances in cost-effective manner.

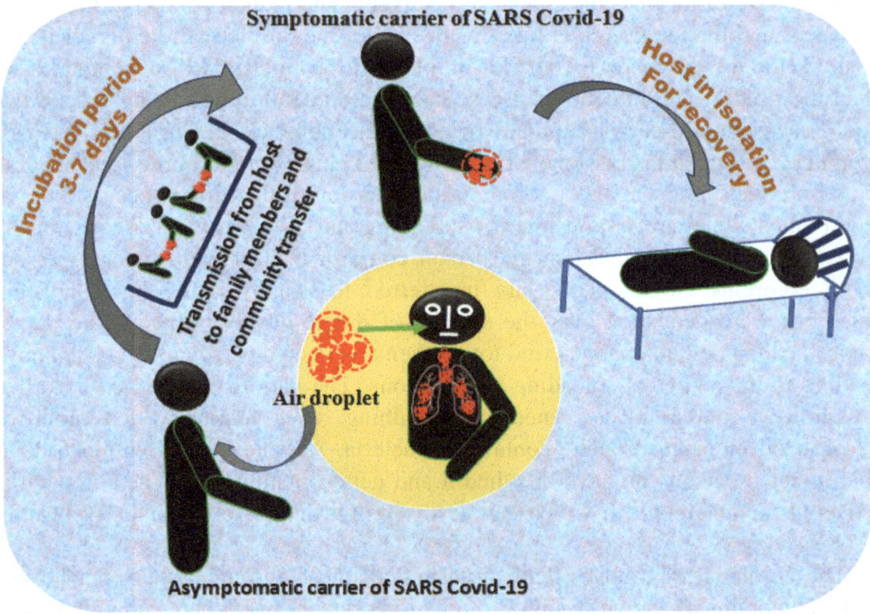

Fig. 2 The path for transmission of COVID-19. Reproduced with permission [7]

4 Preventive Measures

The suspected and confirmed patients of COVID should take treatment in selected hospitals where there is an effective isolation ward and proper protective measures. The suspected patients should be kept in isolation room and persons who are suffering severely should be kept in intensive care unit as soon as possible. The general or preliminary treatment includes best rest, regular monitoring of heart rate, pulse, blood pressure, respiratory rate, oxygen saturation, etc. In the current development, personal protective measures like wearing masks and protective non-woven cloth are used to filter the particles in air to block the droplets, blood, body fluids, secretion, etc. The medical masks were typically made up of from the non-woven layer consisting of functional wet resistant layer, melt-blown non-woven layer, and skin-friendly spun-bonded non-woven layer. The level of filtration of ordinary materials or masks can reach up to 85% so to certify hundred percent filtration performance of medicated mask electrets treatment is necessary [8]. The percentage efficiency of filtration can be reached upto 95% after the effective electrets treatment. The trapped objects like bacteria, viruses, and aerosols are negatively charged which will be blocked by creating electrical field carried out by airflow through positively charge fibers [9]. The effectiveness of mask depends on proper usage and handling, improper usages and touch could increase the probability of transmission of pathogens [10]. By keeping this in mind researchers and R&D department should functionalized the filtration system by adding some of the effective nanomaterials or organic precursor and producing the reusable and recyclable viruses inactivating devices. As a result, it can mitigate the effect of risk being infected by direct and secondary vectors.

There were variety of new ideas, methods, and development in the area of advanced active material that serves as disinfect materials and surface interest. Currently, the advancement of nanotechnology provides an effective pathway for controlling the transmission of contaminated viruses through the proper uses of mask coated with the nanomaterials. Recently variety of nanomaterial has been used for the coating purpose on fibers and non-woven fabrics used for making the mask which is typically applied for face protective measures. For the embedding and coating of fibers and fabrics various inorganic material, organic material and composite materials can be used as advanced functional material. Metal oxide nanoparticles play an important role in the effective coating agent because of its unique physicochemical properties like small particles size, large specific surface area which acts as barriers in between the surface and microorganism. Because of this property a variety of metal oxide nanoparticles like silver (Ag), copper (Cu), titanium (Ti), gold (Au), and zinc (Zn) have been introduced as antiviral agents. The infections of viruses travel mainly via four mechanism, i.e., attachment, penetration, replication, and budding. Whereas, nanoparticle contains three interactive stages (1) linking of connecting to the virus and constraining the attachment of virus in to the cell, (2) production of highly active oxygen which have capabilities of adhering into the wall and destroy the function of proteins and nucleic acid, and (3) inhibiting

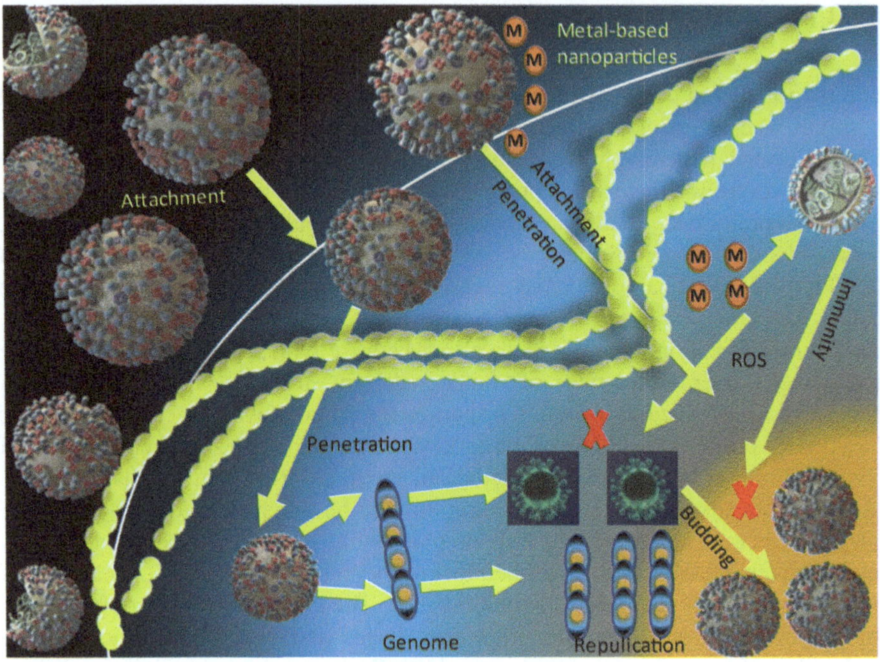

Fig. 3 Schematic representation of antiviral mechanism and metal oxide nanoparticles. Reprint with permission [2]

the budding and spreading of viruses [2]. The schematic representation of antiviral mechanism and metal oxide is shown in Fig. 3.

In spite of metal oxide nanoparticle the organic precursor can also play a vital role for the antiviral coating over the surface of fibers and fabric materials. The organic materials not only kill the pathogen by reaction on the surface proteins or nucleic acid, but it also destroys the further growth of pathogens. On the basis antimicrobial function organic material can be classified into antiviral and photodynamic antiviral materials. Many synthetic and natural organic compounds have intrinsic antiviral properties which lead to virus inactivation due to their chemical structure. Textiles materials provide suitable pathways for the transfer and rapid growth of microbes which causes several deadly diseases, unpleasant odors, declaration and reduces the life span of textile. To protect the transmission of pathogens from textiles to human host, much research has been focussed on the development of new organic material. Various types of chemicals, including quaternary ammonium salts [11], chitosan [12], *N*-halamine, etc., [13] have been developed to produce antibacterial textiles. *N*-halamine is well-established synthetic organic materials well known for its antibacterial activity enabling its deployment for antibacterial fiber modification [14]. *N*-halamine derivatives compound contain multiple nitrogen–halogen covalent polar bonds (NdX), acting as a medium to inactivate microbes rapidly by means of oxidative halogen. On the basis of chemical formula or structure *N*-halamine are classified into three types i.e., (amine *N*-halamine, amide *N*-halamine, and imide *N*-halamine), respectively, as shown in Fig. 4. Due to the existence of the electron/withdrawing donating and electron-withdrawing groups in the chemical groups, their thermal stabilities and antibacterial actions are different which can be predicted by opposite factors [14]. NdX bond can be reduced to NdH, and vice-versa during the course microbe removal which is also a reversible phenomenon. The *N*-halamine containing the reactive agents can attach onto fibers through covalent linkages which confer the durable antibacterial activity on textiles. A series of cyclic *N*-halamine epoxides was successfully synthesized and coated over the surface of fibers (cotton and polyester fabrics) by using pad-dry-cure techniques shown in Fig. 5a, b. Sun and co-workers [15] introduced s-triazine-based *N*-halamine, 2-amino-4-chloro-6-hydroxy-s-triazine (Fig. 5c) has been regarded as a vital reactive agent having the ability to bind with several chemicals containing hydroxyl and amine group which can decrease the damage to physical and mechanical properties of fabrics caused by high temperature during the curing process. Ren et al. [14] demonstrated a non-woven *N*-halamine coated stable and non-volatile fabrics with extremely high antibacterial activity which reduces seven times infection rate by killing the viruses in shorter period of time, disrupting its genetic and replication capabilities. Hydrophilicity of surfaces also plays a crucial role for antiviral activity which restricts the effectiveness of coating. Organic materials are also used for the transforming hydrophilicity surface to the hydrophobic by coating with suitable organic materials. In order to obtain hydrophobic surfaces, the organic chemists or researcher has developed a number of organic materials. In view of this Jayanta et al. [16] synthesized linear or branched hydrophobic *N*,*N*-dodecyl methyl polyethylenimines (PEIs) and tested its antiviral activity hostile to influenza virus which kills the influenza viruses, *Escherichia coli,* and aureus with 100% efficiency within few minutes. The organic materials are also used for the assembling of virus mimic which can easily interact with the receptor and inhibits the attacks of virus to the host cells.

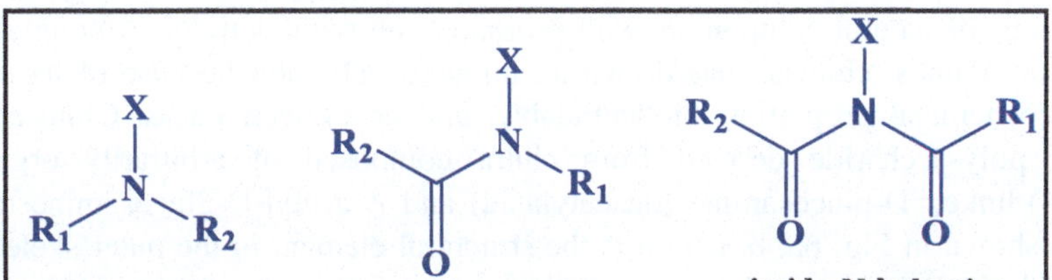

Fig. 4 Chemical structure of different *N*-halamine

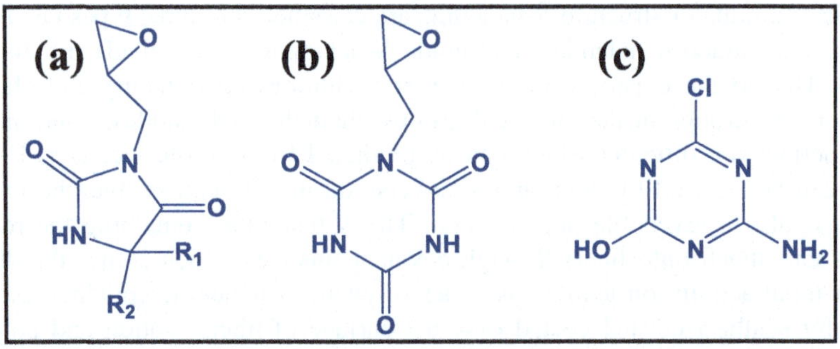

Fig. 5 **a**, **b** Chemical structures of substituted cyclic *N*-halamine epoxides and **c** chemical structure of 2-amino-4-chloro-6-hydroxy-s-triazine

A variety of *N*-halamine containing vinyl group were synthesized and grafted over textile in presence of inhibitors. These chemical compounds are classified into two categories: cyclic and acyclic halamines based on their chemical structure. Majority of cyclic *N*-halamines owe their origin to 5,5-dimethylhydantoin or 2,2,6,6-tetramethyl-4-piperidino reacting with vinyl group such as allyl bromide, acryloyl chloride, methacrylic chloride, and 4-vinylbenzyl chloride. The N-halamine monomer 3-(4′-vinylbenzyl)-5,5-dimethylhydantoin was implemented on the surface of polyester fibers as thin films via surface polymerization with the help of cetylmethylammonium bromide cationic surfactant. In a similar work cotton fabrics impregnated with 2,2,6,6-Tetramethylpiperidinyl acrylate through electron beam radiation was found to be more efficient than conventional techniques without involvement of additional initiators. In line with the development of Kevlar fabric and cellulose via impregnation of acyclic *N*-halamines, acrylamide (AM), and methacrylamide using free radical polymerization yielding comparable biocidal and durable outputs similar to cyclic halamines. However, acyclic halamine are inferior in terms of storage stability and undergo easy hydrolysis compared to bare cyclic counterparts.

In addition to above-synthesized compounds with specific structure, there are numerous of natural compounds with prominent antiviral activity. Among all natural compounds, chitosan has drawn an immense attention because of its unique physicochemical properties, biodegradable, and cost-effectiveness. Chitosan is a linear polysaccharide derived from chitin composed of arbitrarily organized β-(1-4)-linked D-glucosamine (deacetylated) and *N*-acetyl-D-glucosamine (acetylated) shown in Fig. 6a, b. Chitin is the structural element in the outer skeleton of shellfish, including crab, lobster, and shrimp and cell walls of fungi [17] also the second most found polysaccharide following cellulose. The end applications of chitosan depend upon their characteristics like polymer turbidity of polymeric solution, deacetylation degree, and molecular weight [18, 19]. The deacetylation degree is determined by various physical and chemical techniques, i.e., infrared spectroscopy (FTIR), potentiometric titration, along with cutting-edge methods like

^{1}H liquid state and solid state ^{13}C-NMR. The steric exclusion chromatography employing viscometer along with light scattering detector is used to calculate the average molar weight of chitosan [20]. Previously, the complexity in their chemical structure, difficulty in extraction, and insolubility in aqueous solution restrict its application. But nowadays enormous research has been done with chitosan to their practical application in the field of agriculture to fight against fungal infection, pharmaceutical industry, paint industries, biosensor, and energy storage devices, etc. the quality of chitosan depends upon the source of origination of chitin and its method of isolation. The chemical structure of chitosan is presented in Fig. 6a, b.

In spite of all the above application, it has been also used as antiviral coating agent. Md. Ibrahim et al. [21] have studied the antiviral activities of chitosan @ aloe vera modified cotton woven fabric using citric acid cross-linking agent while using the pad-dry-cute method. The existence of the composite over the surface of cotton fabric has been confirmed by the FTIR and SEM techniques. The results of 2 g/l chitosan and 2 g/l aloe vera combinations (composite materials) on cotton fabric have noteworthy antimicrobial inhabitance against *staphylococcus aureus* gram-positive bacteria. Bacteria were reduced by 81% when it is treated with composite material which is greater than the 6 g/l individually treated result. He et al. [22] also demonstrated the antiviral activities of chitosan materials by synthesizing synthesized 6-deoxy-6-bromo-*N*-phthaloyl chitosan. They have additionally reported that chitosan and its derivatives show an excellent antiviral activity. An optimum derivative concentration developed electrospun nanofibrous chitosan to investigate the capability to kill pathogens which reflected a broad spectrum of highly efficient antiviral ability. Pyrazole-based organic compound show a great attention toward the pharmacological assets such as antiviral, anticancer, antimicrobial, antiinflammatory, anti-prostate cancer, herbicidal, and insecticidal properties. Based on the above-said properties Ahmed Nada and

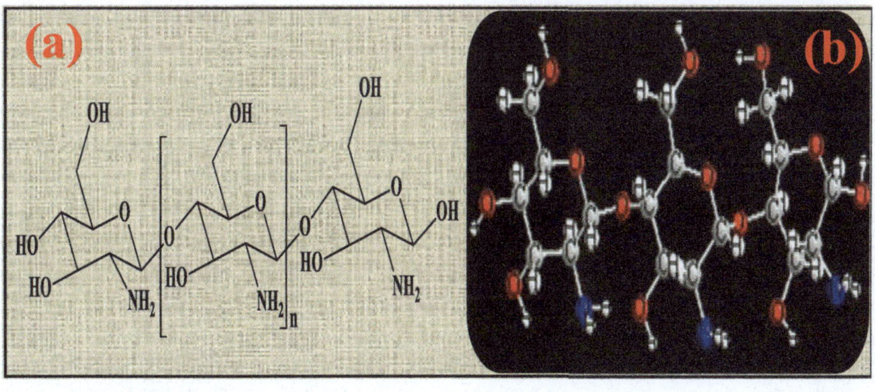

Fig. 6 1D and 3D chemical structure of chitosan

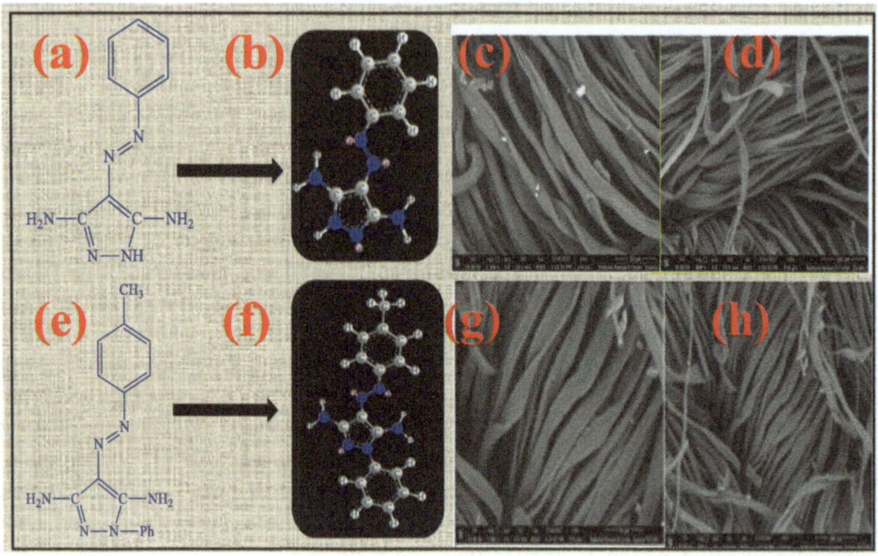

Fig. 7 **a, b, e and f** 1D and 3D structure of pyrazole derivatives, **c** and **d** SEM magnification images of untreated fabrics and **g** and **h** for the treated fabrics. Reprint with permission [23]

co-workers [23] synthesized pyrazole-based compounds and were encapsulated into liposomal chitosan emulsion for textile finishing. The cotton fabrics employed citric acid cross-linker along with treatment in solution-based depolymerized chitosan. The chemical modification of cotton was investigated by infrared spectroscopy analysis. The mechanical strength and retention properties of fabric were investigated by reporting the tensile strength values. The antimicrobial activity of treated cotton fabrics was tested hostile to bacterial strains *E. coli* ATCC 8379 and *S. aureus* ATCC. The chemical structure of pyrazole derivatives and images of untreated and treated fabrics are enlisted in Fig. 7a–h.

The quaternary ammonium salts (QAS) are the ionic compound containing quaternary nitrogen, four alkyl or aryl groups and one anionic ion such as chloride or bromide. The amphiphilicity of polymer is found to be an important factor affecting their antimicrobial performances and hemolytic activity. Among all alkyl groups, one should be of long chain having at least eight hydrocarbon chains which can be treated as hydrophobic group [24]. The chemical structure of various QAS is shown in Fig. 8a, b. Because of the presence of hydrophobic group in the quaternary ammonium salts, it has been explored as a potential source for the antimicrobial function. The risk factor of transmission of infectious diseases in hospital can be reduced by the use of ideal antimicrobial textile which inhibits the growth of microorganism and killing the pathogens. Marini et al. [25] synthesized antimicrobial hybrid coating (organic–inorganic) containing ammonium quaternary salts using tetraethoxysilane and triethoxysilane terminated poly(ethylene glycol)-block-poly(ethylene) followed by sol–gel techniques They have tested

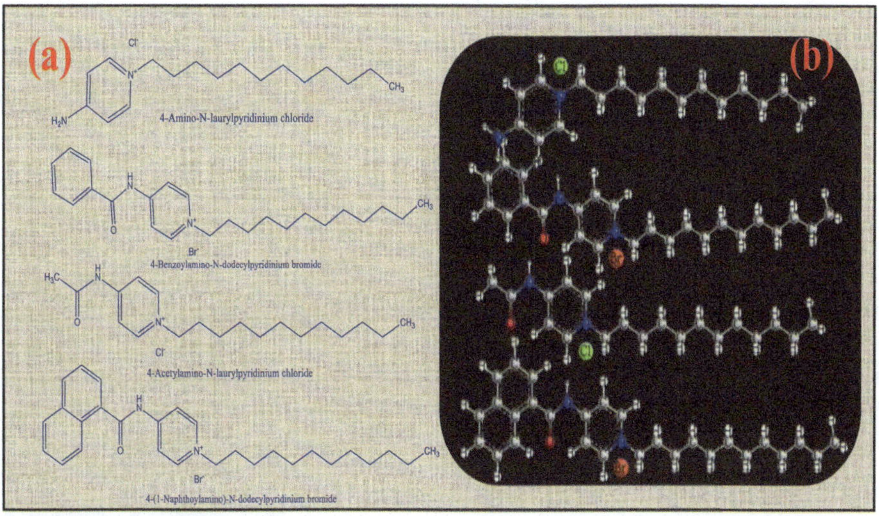

Fig. 8 **a** Chemical structure of various QAS and **b** 3D structure

antimicrobial activity of the coated films against both ram negative and gram-positive bacteria. After 48 h of contact the viable count of bacteria decreases of 96.4% and 99.1% of *E. coli* and *S. aureus*. The stability of the antibacterial activity of coated films was confirmed through repeated washing with saline solution at 37 °C.

5 Photodynamic Antiviral Materials

Photodynamic antiviral materials are generally used for killing the selective pathogens by producing the reactive oxygen species in presence of light. The photodynamic antiviral activity of materials is eco-friendly and safe for the environment by accomplish efficient broad spectrum and long-acting killing of pathogens. On the basis of all said properties it has been widely in the preparation of biological protection materials. Richard et al. [26] demonstrated anti-infective benefits of bulk thermoplastic polymer films containing ~1 wt% zinc-tetra(4-*N*-methylpyridyl) porphine ($ZnTMPyP_4^+$), having antimicrobial activities by creating the singlet oxygen in presence of visible light as shown in Fig. 9. This polymer is having ability to incapacitating both bacteria and viruses with rates of 99.89 and 99.95%, within the exposure of light for 60 min. The use of photodynamic materials in the fibers acts as life-time photosensitizer to killing microorganism by producing reactive oxygen species. They have reported their materials and method are safer and sustainable due to the reliance on visible light and oxygen availability only. Mosinger et al. [27] prepared a stable photoactive polystyrene nanoparticle

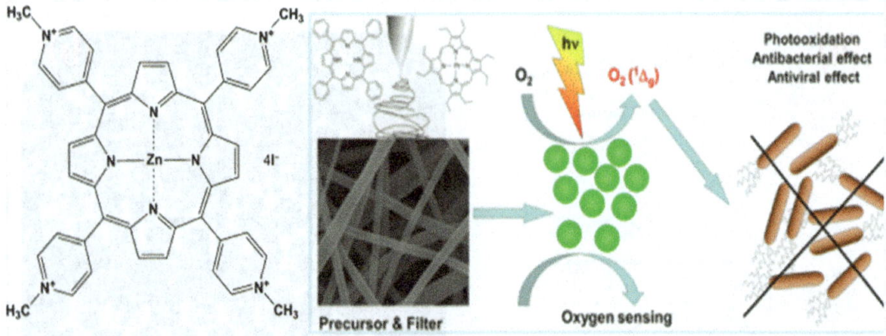

Fig. 9 a Chemical structure of the photosensitizer Zinc-tetra(4-methylpyridyl) porphine (ZnTMPyP4+) and **b** schematic representation of Pt-OEP [26, 29]

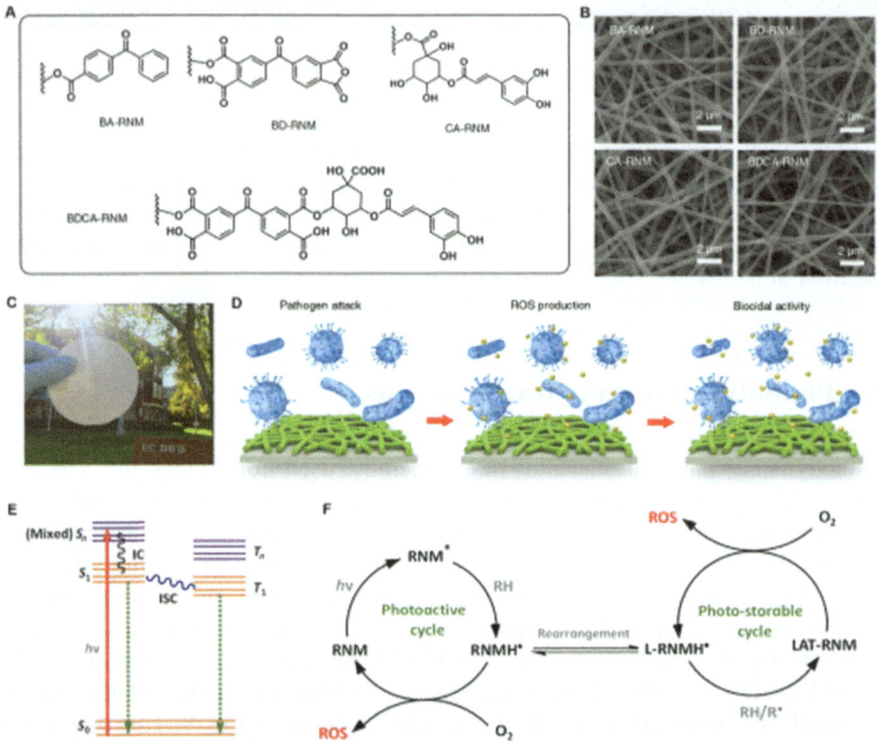

Fig. 10 a Chemical structure of BA-RNM, BD-RNM, CA-RNM, and BDCA-RNM. **b** Microscopic architecture of various RNM samples. **c** Optical photograph of the BDCA-RNM sample. **d** Schematic demonstration of the biocidal functions of RNMs by releasing ROS. **e** Jablonski diagrams representing the singlet excitation and following ISC to triplet. **f** Proposed mechanism for the photoactive and photo-storable biocidal cycles. Reprint with permission [28]

from sulfonated electrospun polystyrene nanofibers membrane with encapsulated 5,10,15,20-tetraphenylporphyrin (TPP) or platinum octaethylporphyrin (Pt-OEP). The nanoparticle and TPP are strongly antibacterial activities and can be employed for photooxidation of external substrate grounded on photogenerated single oxygen. The polyethylene nanofibers membrane was synthesized using electrospun method for encapsulating the photosensitizer. The nanofibers membrane constrained the growth of bacteria and viruses with an high efficiency of more than 99% when exposed to visible light, additionally a simultaneous bacterial inhibition in both light and dark condition instantly was observed. This necessitates an apt solution to address the efficiency in dyssophotic environment. Sun et al. [28] prepared nanofibers membrane endowing superior antiviral activities guided by day-light via electrospun method as shown in Fig. 10. Based on ROS yield the membrane show excellent killing both for virus and bacterias. Additionally, the membrane was also successful in retaining their biological activities in presence of sunlight. The ability of the membrane was further tested in bioprotective equipment to test their effectiveness on killing pathogens and aerosols. The results confirm a killing efficiency of 100% establishing their potential as filtration membrane even efficient than the commercial ones.

6 Conclusion

The main objective of this chapter is to highlight the recent developed or progress in the field of therapeutic applications. A broad range of properties exhibited by organic materials including chitosan and its composite, *N*-halamine, and quaternary ammonium salts which have application prospects in the therapeutic need as the preventive measures to fight against novel coronaviruses. Currently, available antiviral personal protective devices like sanitizer, hand wash, gloves, and face mask. Especially, face mask has drawn a great attention for the scientific community and academician for the development of new and advanced mask. The maximum masks available in market are unable to protect sufficiently the filter of tiny aerogels containing viruses. The microbes get involved to be filtering materials which penetrate via the moist mask increases the risk of infections. This chapter deals with current advances in antiviral agents, and recently developed method used for the preparation of protective materials results in improving the antiviral coating. The advanced organic materials are introduced to the surface of masks lead to increase efficiency of antiviral capabilities of masks which reduces the risk of cross-infection at the course of handling. A variety of organic materials have been incorporated and explored which are the integrable into the face masks. The mechanistic approach and the physical and chemical properties of fabrics are also incorporated after introduction of organic material. Here we have also discussed their percentage of effectiveness compared to the bare cloth or fabrics. As concluding remarks, chapter focusses on current shortcoming in personal protective kit running to the lack of enough comfort high efficiency, safety, and intelligence. The serious drawbacks can solve by developing a new engineered material adapted with the face mask, skin, and body which control the unwanted affects and make it ease for continuous use.

Acknowledgments All the authors are thankful for their institutional support.

Author Contributions All the authors have equally contributed in data collection, drafting, editing, or revising the articles to make it publishable format.

Conflict of Interests Authors declare no conflict of interest in this work.

References

1. Weiss C, Carriere M, Fusco L, Capua I, Regla-Nava JA, Pasquali M, Scott JA, Vitale F, Unal MA, Mattevi C (2020) Toward nanotechnology-enabled approaches against the COVID-19 pandemic. ACS Nano 14(6):6383–6406
2. Zhou J, Hu Z, Zabihi F, Chen Z, Zhu M (2020) Progress and perspective of antiviral protective material. Adv Fiber Mater 2:123–139
3. Lovato A, de Filippis C (2020) Clinical presentation of COVID-19: a systematic review focusing on upper airway symptoms. Ear Nose Throat J 99(6):569–576
4. Wang J, Tang K, Feng K, Lv W (2020) High temperature and high humidity reduce the transmission of COVID-19. Available at SSRN 3551767
5. Mallapaty S Why does the coronavirus spread so easily between people? Nature. https://doi.org/10.1038/d41586-020-00660-x
6. Bai Y, Yao L, Wei T, Tian F, Jin D-Y, Chen L, Wang M (2020) Presumed asymptomatic carrier transmission of COVID-19. JAMA 323:1406–1407
7. Rocky MMH, Bhuyan MAH, Khan R, Akhtar S A simple homemade cloth mask for mass people in Covid-19: salt-starching treatment on fabric for better bioaerosol filtration efficiency. https://doi.org/10.13140/RG.2.2.26003.91681
8. Iwata M, Tanizaki H, Fujii H, Endo Y, Fujisawa A, Tanioka M, Miyachi Y, Kabashima K (2015) Contact urticaria due to a face mask coated with disinfectant liquid spray. Acta Derm Venereol 95:628–629
9. Winski TA, Mueller WA, Graveling RA (2019) If the mask fits: facial dimensions and mask performance. Int J Ind Ergon 72:308–310
10. Li Y, Leung P, Yao L, Song Q, Newton E (2006) Antimicrobial effect of surgical masks coated with nanoparticles. J Hosp Infect 62:58–63
11. Lundin JG, Coneski PN, Fulmer PA, Wynne JH (2014) Relationship between surface concentration of amphiphilic quaternary ammonium biocides in electrospun polymer fibers and biocidal activity. React Funct Polym 77:39–46
12. Kim SS, Lee J (2014) Antibacterial activity of polyacrylonitrile–chitosan electrospun nanofibers. Carbohyd Polym 102:231–237
13. Ren T, Dormitorio TV, Qiao M, Huang T-S, Weese J (2018) *N*-halamine incorporated antimicrobial nonwoven fabrics for use against avian influenza virus. Vet Microbiol 218:78–83
14. Ren X, Jiang Z, Liu Y, Li L, Fan X (2016) *N*-halamines as antimicrobial textile finishes. In: Antimicrobial textiles. Woodhead publishing, pp 125–140

15. Braun M, Sun Y (2004) Antimicrobial polymers containing melamine derivatives. I. Preparation and characterization of chloromelamine-based cellulose. J Polym Sci Part A: Polym Chem 42:3818–3827
16. Haldar J, An D, de Cienfuegos LA, Chen J, Klibanov AM (2006) Polymeric coatings that inactivate both influenza virus and pathogenic bacteria. Proc Natl Acad Sci 103:17667–17671
17. Cheung RCF, Ng TB, Wong JH, Chan WY (2015) Chitosan: an update on potential biomedical and pharmaceutical applications. Mar Drugs 13:5156–5186
18. Nwe N, Furuike T, Tamura H (2014) Isolation and characterization of chitin and chitosan from marine origin. Adv Food Nutr Res 72:1–15
19. Galed G, Miralles B, Paños I, Santiago A, Heras Á (2005) *N*-deacetylation and depolymerization reactions of chitin/chitosan: influence of the source of chitin. Carbohyd Polym 62:316–320
20. Younes I, Rinaudo M (2015) Chitin and chitosan preparation from marine sources. Struct Prop Appl Mar Drugs 13:1133–1174
21. Mondal MIH, Saha J (2019) Antimicrobial, UV resistant and thermal comfort properties of chitosan-and Aloe vera-modified cotton woven fabric. J Polym Environ 27:405–420
22. He X, Xing R, Liu S, Qin Y, Li K, Yu H, Li P (2019) The improved antiviral activities of amino-modified chitosan derivatives on Newcastle virus. Drug Chem Toxicol 1–6
23. Nada A, Al- M, Soliman AA, Rashwan GM, Eldawy THA, Hassan AAE, Sayed GH (2018) Pyrazole-based compounds in chitosan liposomal emulsion for antimicrobial cotton fabrics. Int J Biol Macromol 107:585–594
24. Sun G (2011) Antibacterial textile materials for medical applications. In: Functional textiles for improved performance, protection and health. Woodhead publishing, pp 360–375
25. Marini M, Bondi M, Iseppi R, Toselli M, Pilati F (2007) Preparation and antibacterial activity of hybrid materials containing quaternary ammonium salts via sol–gel process. Eur Polymer J 43:3621–3628
26. Peddinti BS, Scholle F, Ghiladi RA, Spontak RJ (2018) Photodynamic polymers as comprehensive anti-infective materials: staying ahead of a growing global threat. ACS Appl Mater Interfaces 10:25955–25959
27. Henke P, Kirakci K, Kubát P, Fraiberk M, Forstová J, Mosinger J (2016) Antibacterial, antiviral, and oxygen-sensing nanoparticles prepared from electrospun materials. ACS Appl Mater Interfaces 8:25127–25136
28. Si Y, Zhang Z, Wu W, Fu Q, Huang K, Nitin N, Ding B, Sun G Daylight-driven rechargeable antibacterial and antiviral nanofibrous membranes for bioprotective applications. Sci Adv. https://doi.org/10.1126/sciadv.aar5931
29. Adeli H, Khorasani MT, Parvazinia M (2019) Wound dressing based on electrospun PVA/chitosan/starch nanofibrous mats: fabrication, antibacterial and cytocompatibility evaluation and in vitro healing assay. Int J Biol Macromol 122:238–254

Chapter 6
Material Aspects for Detection and Monitoring

Priyanka Mukherjee and Mamata Mohapatra

1 Introduction

The widespread pandemic caused due to novel coronavirus is not the first of its kind in this millennium. Early 2003 has witnessed the outbreak of SARS-COVID in parts of China. With a fatality rate of 10% and more than 8000 registered cases, societies and economies were severely impacted, and within a few months, the epidemic was unparalleled to the last outbreak. The spread of the virus was restricted to a small perimeter along with a high-alert warning to limit the consumption of proteins from exotic and endangered animals [1–5]. The epidemic caused by the coronavirus resurfaced in December 2019 in Wuhan city of China.

Since individuals of all ages are at risk for infection and the virus is several communicable, it was proclaimed to be a Public Health Emergency of International Concern by the WHO on 30 January 2020 [6, 7]. Figure 1 depicts the countries having highest number of COVID-19 tests across the world. With the increasing number cases with clear symptoms, asymptomatic cases are also increasing rapidly. On surveying the number of diagnostic tests conducted globally as of August 2020 India ranked first worldwide followed by the UK and South Africa. Rapid economic growth in various parts of China led to massive upsurge in demand of animal proteins. Lack of proper bio-safety measures with overloaded cages and jammed wet markets led to limping of the virus from animals to humans.

The extent of transmission by such cases remains unknown, and hence, they contribute substantially to community transfers. Figure 2 shows the modes of transmission of the virus to human colonial zones. As on 28 August 2020, 24.5 million active cases of the coronavirus were confirmed in 213 countries globally

P. Mukherjee (✉) · M. Mohapatra
CSIR-Institute of Minerals and Materials Technology, Bhubaneswar, Odisha 751013, India
e-mail: priyanka.m@immt.res.in

M. Mohapatra
e-mail: mamata@immt.res.in

M. Mohapatra et al. (eds.), *COVID-19 Pandemic*, Materials Horizons: From Nature to Nanomaterials, https://doi.org/10.1007/978-981-16-4372-9_6

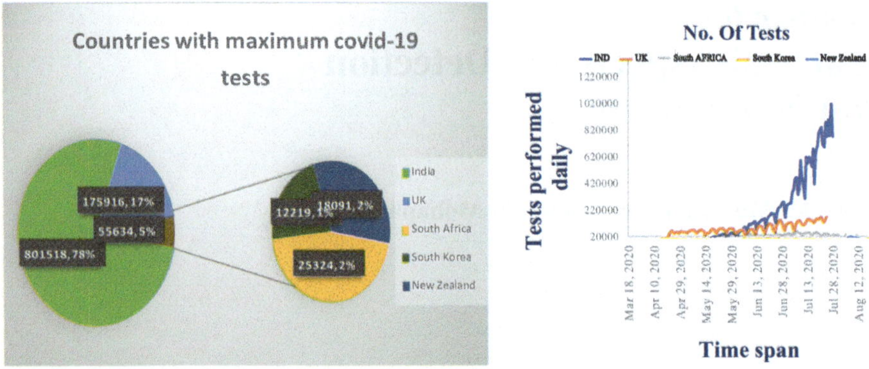

Fig. 1 Countries having highest number of COVID-19 tests across the world

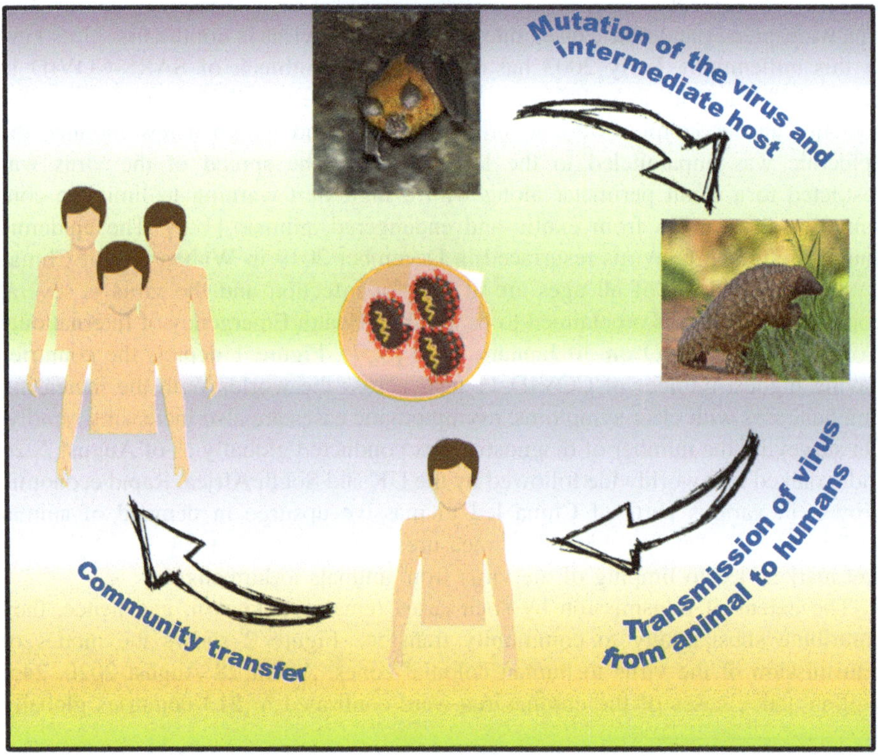

Fig. 2 Modes of transmission of the virus to human colonial zones

along with a death toll of 832,000 [8–10]. One of the many reasons for transmission of SARS-CoV-2 globally is the lack of public awareness about a safe perimeter. Community transfers occurred when a healthy person being unaware of the fact, crossed paths with a virus infected person. The major challenge in controlling COVID-19 is the massive percentage of infected people. However, early detection, precise diagnosis and management of severely infected cases are the key points in combating the current situation.

For highly accurate assessment of the cases, a better understanding of the test probability of serology, qRT-PCR and radiological testing and the efficiency of available treatment options are required. Literatures report that a major fraction of people infected by the corona virus had fever at the time of diagnosis whereas the other fraction had common symptoms like cough, fatigue and breathlessness [11–17]. Many of these symptoms being similar to other respiratory infections. Thus, diagnostic tests specific to this infection are urgently required to confirm suspected cases, screen patients and conduct virus surveillance. Herein, the authors focus on the various available diagnostic techniques and their material aspects that make these test platforms highly selective and specific to the detection of SARS-COVID-19.

2 Types of Viable Detection Techniques

Structural elucidation of the virus and critical analysis of the composition are the keys to accurate diagnosis and detection. Although the protein and genetic coding of SARS-CoV- 2 have been identified so far, its response to the host cell continues to be under trials. Figure 3 shows the various types of sensors for preliminary diagnosis of SARS-COVID-19. Preliminary diagnosis and screening of COVID-19 have been carried out by CT scans and nucleic acid testing. Various types of sensors like electrochemical biosensors, optical biosensors, thermal biosensors and piezoelectric biosensors have been widely explored to diagnose viral genomes.

Nanotechnology has advanced treatment and therapeutic procedures of medical science by several folds. Different strategies based on nanotechnology have been developed to detect and diagnose COVID-19 by methods like POC, RT-PCR, RT-LAMP, NTS and such others. It has helped to create effective treatment methods by improvement in areas ranging from targeted drug delivery to the production of inexpensive and scalable detection methods. Nanosensors have been reported to detect ultra-low viral load in patients which implies that accurate and rapid diagnosis is possible even before the symptoms appear substantially. DNA sequencing methods such as Oxford nanopore sequencing method and Illumina method have been applied to nearly 104 isolated SARS-CoV-2 viral strains [18–21]. The best weapon to combat COVID-19 pandemic is continuous R&D in nanotechnology to diagnose, treat the virus with advanced and modified instruments and in areas of medical sciences to develop vaccines and antibodies that would engulf and destroy the virus [22–27]. The currently developed techniques for detection and diagnosis of COVID-19 have been discussed Table 1.

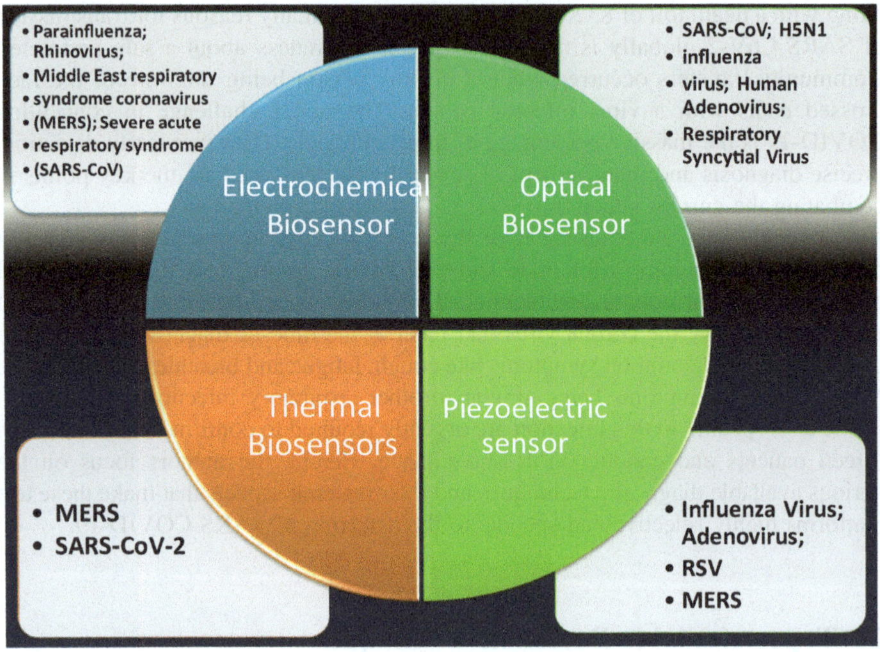

Fig. 3 Various types of sensors for preliminary diagnosis of SARS-COVID-19

Table 1 Types of viable detection techniques based on nanotechnology

S. No.	Detection methods	Advantage	Limitation	References
1	ID NOW	Specificity of the assay is 100%	Lack in sensitivity while diagnosing weakly positive samples	Stephanie et al. [28]
2	Xpert Xpress point-of-care assay (Cepheid GeneXpert systems) for targeting SARS-CoV-2 E-gene and N2-gene in three medical laboratories in the Netherlands	The assay can detect SARS-CoV-2 with a LOD of 8.26 copies/mL in all three laboratories		Femke et al. [29]
3	Xpert Xpress test for targeting SARS-CoV-2 E-gene and N2-gene	LOD of 100 copies/mL	Lowest LOD (100 copies/mL)	Wei et al. [30]

(continued)

Table 1 (continued)

S. No.	Detection methods	Advantage	Limitation	References
4	Amplicon sequencing	Cost-effective, highly sensitive suitable for samples with low viral load	Ultra-modern instrumentation with skilled man power disability to sequence highly diverse or recombinant viruses	Xiao et al. [31]
5	One-step nested real-time RT-PCR (OSN-qRT-PCR) assay for targeting SARS-CoV-2 ORF1ab and N genes	The sensitivity of the assay was 1 copy/test and tenfold higher than that of commercial qRT-PCR assay	Laboratory cross-contamination, which may lead to false positive results	Ji et al. [32]
6	ddPCR for SARS-CoV-2 RNA detection	Highly increased sensitivity and accuracy. Nearly a 40% increase in precision and 47% for RT-PCR to 94% and 95% for ddPCR	Expensive than qRT-PCR and requires dedicated instruments and consumables	Suo et al. [33]
7	LAMP primers targeting the 5′ region of the ORF1a and N genes of SARS-CoV-2 and detected by a visual, colorimetric RT-LAMP	The colorimetric RT-LAMP analysis was 100% consistent with RT-PCR results across a range of Cq values, and matches RT-PCR on-field and point-of-care tests		Zhang et al. [34]
8	Colorimetric test based on gold nanoparticles (AuNPs) with thiol-modified antisense oligonucleotides (ASOs) targeting the SARS-CoV-2 N-gene	The limit of detection (LOD) was found to be 0.18 ng/μL of SARS-CoV-2 viral load	Complex pre-treatment steps, costlier than qRT-PCR techniques	Parikshit et al. [35]
9	QIAstat-Dx Respiratory SARS-CoV-2 Panel for SARS-CoV-2 detection	More sensitivity to RT-PCR with a LOD at 1000 copies/mL		Benoit et al. [36]

3 Material Approach of Various Diagnostic Methods

3.1 Point-Of-Care Tests

Diagnostic methods based on application of nanomaterials have been proven suitable for rapid and accurate detection of SARS-CoV-2. Diagnostic tests that are performed at the site of infected patients are called point-of-care test. In these techniques, the test samples are not required to be sent to any laboratory and are simple to use methods. The advantages of POC tests are speed of diagnosis, simplified user interface like membrane strips, push buttons, cost-effectiveness and ease of availability. Different types of POC tests can be classified into following groups as nucleic acid amplification (molecular) tests, antigen tests and serological tests. Out of many POC-based diagnostic methods where detection for SARS-CoV-2 is being carried out, the lateral flow method is a very popular technique based on antibody/antigen techniques [37–42]. It is a care point test where a paper like membrane strip is used which contains two flow channels coated on the strip. One of the channels contains Au NPs antibodies and the other captures the antibody. Figure 4 depicts the working of strip-based antibody/antigen detection technique. Test samples, generally being patient's urine or blood, are collected on the membrane and under the capillary action the protein starts moving across the channels. When the first line moves, the nanoparticle-antibody gold conjugate traps the antigens, and the complex flows across the membrane. On entering the second line, the trapped antibody immobilizes the complex where the red or blue side is visible. Bare Au NPs are red, and the coupled Plasmon causes the solution containing the coupled Au NPs to turn blue.

Another outstanding development in the POC tests is combination of the test with mobile phones. Yang T et al. reported integration of cellular phone with a strip-based PoC testing device along with PCR and LAMP assays. In this technique, a patient can easily test himself by collecting nasal swab samples and the result will be shared by mobile app to the concerned people. Trieu Nguyen also reported 7 integration of a mobile phone app with LAMP assay on a paper-based PoC device where instead of heat denaturation of the nuclei acid, the strands were displaced. The colorimetric reaction is detected on the mobile app specially designed to detect colorimetric changes on paper and the result is shared with the patient a well as medical authorities. These techniques can increase the accessibility of self-quarantined people to avail the tests easily, and due to the combination of PCR and LAMP assays, the chances of false negative tests have also been minimized.

Focusing on the commercially approved devices, an excellent example of widely available mobile molecular POC device for SARS-CoV-2 is Abbott ID NOW. Another example of a larger facility-based POC platforms for SARS-CoV-2 is the Cepheid GeneXpert® Xpress. Both these techniques yield return results in less than an hour's time; however, based on their mechanism of action, these techniques may not detect all active infections. Thus, a positive or a negative test must be confirmed

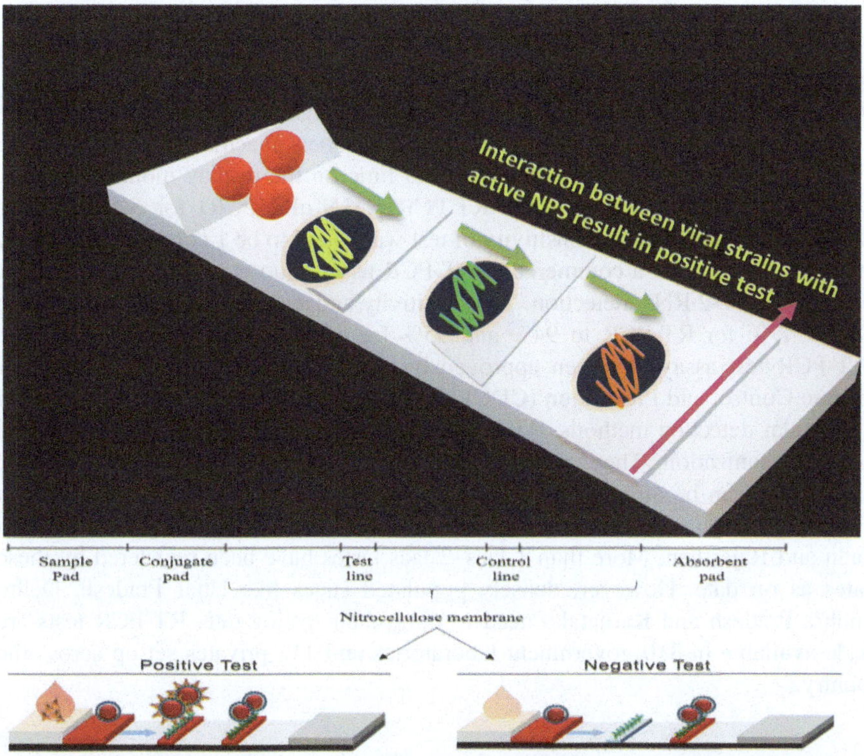

Fig. 4 Mechanism for detection of lateral flow antigen method

further by a PCR test. Hence, in order for accurate and precise detection of SARS-COVID-2 possible, molecular tests are more reliable to diagnose the presence of SARS-CoV-2 infections.

3.2 *RT-PCR*

The next method that has gained gigantic importance in detection of COVID-19 is the quantitative reverse transcription polymerase chain reaction (qRT-PCR) test. This is a method which is highly specific to analysis of swabs from nasopharynx for the presence of virial nucleic acids. Because of the high precision and accuracy in detection results of SARS-CoV-2, for PCR tests, swab samples are collected from nasopharynx and throat where the probable density of the virus is highest. The RNA is then extracted from the swab by treating it with chemical agents so that the fats and protein layers' dissolve from the RNA. After reverse transcription of the RNA using a specific enzyme into DNA, small fragments of complementary

DNA are added to specific parts of the viral DNA so that they attach themselves to parts of the transcribed DNA if the virus is present. Parts of these fragments are used to build DNA strands for amplification and the rest is used as marker labels. The samples are then placed in RT-PCR machine where cycles are run to produce identical copies of the viral DNA and the marker labels attach themselves releasing a fluorescent dye which is presented as real time on the display monitor. Ji et al. reported one-step nested real-time RT-PCR (OSN-qRT-PCR) for SARS-CoV-2 ORF1ab and N genes. The sensitivity of test was found to be 1 copy/test and nearly ten times higher than a commercial qRT-PCR assay. Suo et al. reported a ddPCR for SARS-CoV-2 RNA detection. The sensitivity and accuracy were increased from 40 and 47% for RT-PCR to 94% and 95% for ddPCR. Out of all the tests, the qRT-PCR test assay has been approved by the (WHO) and the US Centres for Disease Control and Prevention (CDC) [43–45]. Figure 5 depicts the efficiencies of the popular detection methods. RT-PCR tests the only ones validated by the World Health Organization. They are the gold standard in diagnosing COVID-19, and thus, a case can be affirmed by this test. According to recent reports, the highest number of tests in India has been conducted by the states of Maharashtra, Tamil Nadu and Rajasthan. More than 1 lacs–2 lacs testes have been registered by these states as on date. However, densely populated states like Uttar Pradesh, Delhi, Andhra Pradesh and Karnataka need to ramp their testing rate. RT-PCR tests are made available in 310 government laboratories and 111 privates set up across the country.

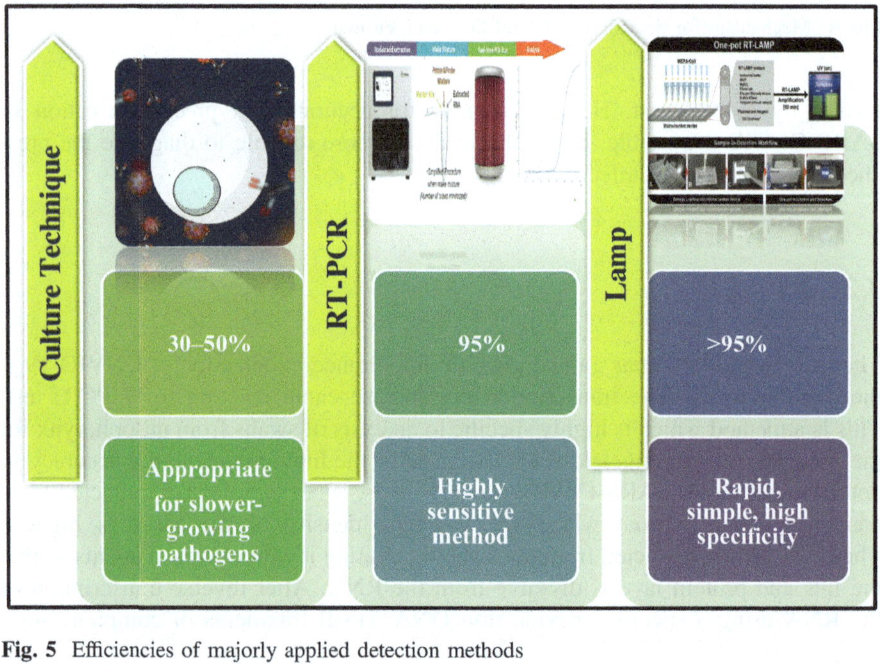

Fig. 5 Efficiencies of majorly applied detection methods

The ICMR has emphasized that the confirmatory test for diagnosis of COVID-19 infection is RT-PCR test of the throat and/or nasal swab, which detects virus at an early stage; hence, RT-PCR tests must be continued vigorously as the principal diagnostic tests. However, with the rapid spread of the pandemic, the test falls behind lacking the required screening capacity and suffers some major limitations like lengthy hours for analysis of test data, use of complex instrumentation, availability of space and requirement of highly skilled and trained personnel's [46].

3.3 Reverse Transcription Loop-Mediated Isothermal Amplification

Despite the rapid diagnosis and accuracy of detection in the above methods, the drawbacks are requirement of highly skilled manpower and the efficacy of detection over larger intervals. Thus, the next method to be discussed in the following section is reverse transcription loop-mediated isothermal amplification (RT-LAMP) assay. It is a single-step process with minimum limitations than QRT-PCR, NTS and other POCs and marches ahead with advantages of being rapid, viable for a wide range of sample types and the use of easily available chemicals that and can be stored at ambient conditions. Yang et al. initially reported an RT-LAMP assay dating back to 2003 for successful detection of SARS-CoV-2 [47–49], and it has been further developed since for highly accurate and speedy diagnosis of COVID-19. The LAMP assay comprises of two sets of inner and outer primer that identify the targeted DNA strand. The components of forward the inner primer are the F2 region and a (F1c) region, which is the complementary of F1 region and the components of the backward inner primer are the B2 region and a (B1c) region. Similarly, the forward outer primer contains (F3) and backward outer primer (B3) has the sequences that are complementary to the sequences of the F3c and B3c regions, respectively. At first, FIP forms complex with targeted DNA at F2 region to form double stranded complex at an optimum temperature of 65 which is then followed by the initiation of DNA synthesis. The F3 primer on binding with F3c displaces FIP complementary strand, and FIP now forms a loop on one end of the DNA which serve as a target to the BIP. The resultant dumbbell-like structure serves as DNA amplification template. In RT-LAMP, reverse transcriptase is added for conversion of RNA to complementary DNA which is then amplified. Nearly 30 min is the estimated time for amplification at a constant 60–65 °C using different primers to detect the N, E and ORF1ab genes, and the results are macroscopically visible by the colour change. In order to enhance the sensitivity further, nanomaterials have been combined with LAMP techniques. Their excellent opto-electronic properties combined with the receptors which are basically biomolecules are highly selective to particular analysts. Recently, LAMP assay has been combined with nanobiosensors (NBS), nanoparticle aided laminar flow (LFB) and such other nano-based platforms for even better detection results. Lamb et al. reported rapid screening LAMP test for COVID-19 sequence in less than 30 min with an LOD of 1.02 fg/reaction using simulated samples. Yu et al. reported iLACO assay for COVID-19 to target on ORF1ab gene, the LOD was about 10 copies of the ORF1ab gene. Wang et al. reported an RT-LAMP assay for COVID-19 where two different one-pot assays, namely a one-pot real-time assay RT-LAMP and one-pot visual RT-LAMP, were tested at an optimized temperature of 59° C, the LOD was 6 copies of nucleic acid. Mohammed et al. reported the method of Penn-RAMP Recombinase polymerase amplification (RPA). This test results in an LOD of 70 copies/reaction. J.P brought et al. reported an integrated RT-LAMP with CRISPR–Cas12 DETECTR technology where the N genes targeted by DETECTR. Assay only detects the SARS-CoV-2 virus, while the E gene-targeted assay detected SARS-CoV-2, SARS-CoV and bat-SL-CoVZC45 viruses. The LOD was 10 copies/ L to 15,000 and 500 copies per L, respectively. The recent development in the RT-LAMP processes has been grouped in Table 2.

4 Role of Nanomaterials in Diagnosis

Viewing the enormous consumption of time in the prevailing conventional diagnostic techniques, there huge urgency to design and fabricate rapid and highly accurate nanosensor for detecting SARS-CoV-2.

Biosensors aided with nanoparticles have emerged as highly attractive and promising detection tools for pathogenic and viral diseases among individuals. In view of the persistent demerits of the conventional detection methods like false negative rates, lack of specificity when compared to other viruses, high time consumption and lower sensitivity, nanomaterials like the quantum dots have been successfully reported and reviewed for their vital therapeutic and diagnostic aspects. On the contrast, such reliable and accurate techniques for the detection of COVID-19 are yet to be developed. Figure 6 depicts the route of action of nanomaterials in supressing the virus.

Nanotechnology has emerged as a breakthrough in advanced detection by including device integration, improved sensing unit, packaging and sensing results of the point-of-care testes which have enhanced the diagnostics via disease management in a personalized manner and the catered to the requirement of the patient. Thus, the need of the hour is to design easy-to-use, fast and more simplistic detection techniques for COVID-19. Magnetic nanoparticles have been reported earlier for their high efficiency in sensory systems. Recently, Zhao et al. reported an alternative route by the use of poly (amino ester) and carboxyl groups (PC)-coated magnetic nanoparticles (pcMNPs) [57]. The synthesized pcMNPs were directly introduced into a RT-PCR reaction initiated resulting in a single step which was the combination of the lysis and binding step. Within 20 min, this technique separates viral RNA from multiple samples and produces 10-copy sensitivity with strong linear correlation between 10 and 105 copies of SARS-CoV-2 pseudovirus particles.

Table 2 Various types of loop-mediated isothermal amplification (LAMP) techniques

S. No	LAMP techniques	Course of the process	LOD	Analysis	References
1	Rapid screening LAMP test	Genetic sequencing of the virus and LAMP Designer 1.15 (Premier Biosoft), accurate identification of swabs from serum, urine, saliva, oropharyngeal and nasopharyngeal with spiked COVID-19 sequence were all correctly identified	> 30 min, limit of detection = 1.02 fg/reaction using simulated samples	Three methods: colour change, fluorescence, and gel electrophoresis	Lamb et al. [50]
2	iLACO assay for COVID-19 (isothermal LAMP-based method for COVID-19) to target on ORF1ab gene	Well-designed RT-LAMP primer set bearing high specificity and can generate high sensitivity and high accuracy in COVID-19 clinical sample test	LOD of iLACO assay is about 10 copies of the ORF1ab gene	SYBR green dye initially used for enhanced fluorescence, which was t replaced by GeneFinder dye with blue light for dilute solution	Yu et al. [51]
3	One-pot RT-LAMP assay for COVID-19	Two different one-pot assays namely one-pot real-time RT-LAMP assay and one-pot visual RT-LAMP assay are tested at optimized temperature of 59° C	LOD = 6 copies of nucleic acid	Fluorescence signal detection was accomplished using a StepOneTM System, while the end-point visual colour changes was realized by using colour indicator	Yu et al. [52]
4	Penn-RAMP	Recombinase polymerase amplification (RPA) process is conducted and after amplification the RPA mixture is blended into LAMP reaction reagents that were pre-loaded in the test tube	70 copies/reaction	–	El-Tholoth et al [53]
5	Integrated RT-LAMP combination of RT-LAMP technology with CRISPR–Cas12 DETECTR technology	The N gene-targeted DETECTR assay only detects the SARS-CoV-2 virus, while the E gene-targeted assay detected SARS-CoV-2, SARS-CoV, and bat-SL-CoVZC45 viruses	10 copies/ L to 15,000 and 500 copies per L, respectively	Visualization of the assay is achieved using a FAM-biotin reporter molecule and lateral flow strips designed to capture labelled nucleic acids	Broughton [54]

(continued)

Table 2 (continued)

S. No	LAMP techniques	Course of the process	LOD	Analysis	References
6	STOP COVID (SHERLOCK testing in one pot for COVID-19)		100 copies per reaction, which was confirmed with 30 trials of the test	Lateral flow strip or fluorescent reporter	Joung et al. [55]
7	mRT-LAMP-LFB	Using two LAMP primer sets, the ORF1ab (opening reading frame 1a/b) and N (nucleoprotein) genes of SARS-CoV-2 were simultaneously amplified in a single-tube using Dye streptavidin coated polymer nanoparticles	12 copies (for each detection target) per reaction	Accumulation of nanoparticles leaded a characteristic crimson band, enabling multiplex analysis of ORF1ab and N gene without instrumentation	Zhu et al. [56]

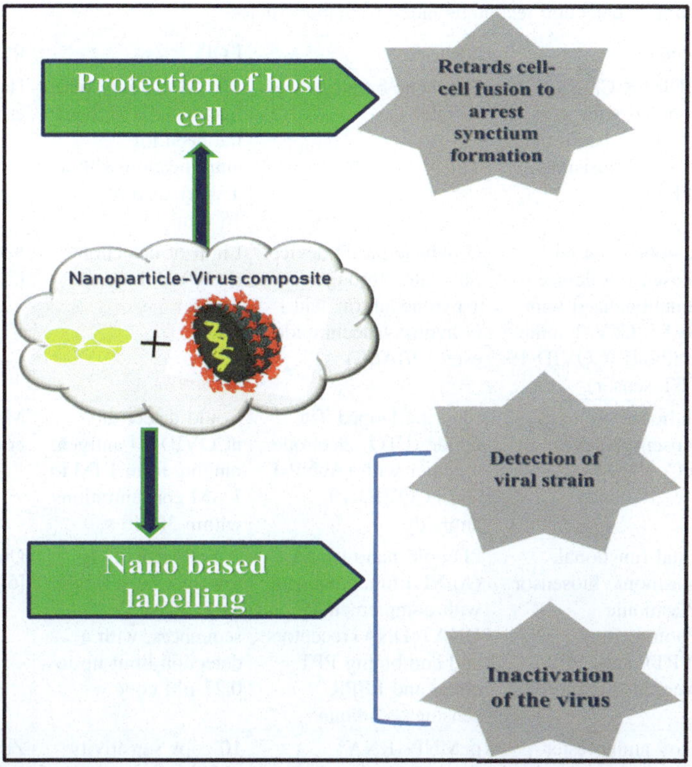

Fig. 6 Route of action of nanomaterials in supressing the virus

This technique was successful in reducing the operational requirements. Table 3 shows various detection technique aided by nanoparticles. Table 3 lists various detection technique aided by nanoparticles.

5 Nanopore Target Sequencing (NTS)

Targeted gene sequencing techniques have become very popular in diagnosis of genetic mutation. These are highly precise, accurate and can detect multiple pathogens. The nanopore target sequence is an advanced version of the existing technique with a capacity to detect nearly 10 different pulmonary viruses in addition to diagnosis of SARS-CoV-2. Targeted gene sequencing techniques have become very popular in the diagnosis of genetic mutation. These are highly precise, accurate and can detect multiple pathogens. The nanopore target sequence is an advanced version of the existing technique with a capacity to detect nearly ten different pulmonary viruses in addition to the diagnosis of SARS-CoV-2. With the aid of

Table 3 Various detection technique aided by nanoparticles

S. No.	Method	NP used	LOD	References
1	CRISPR-Chip coupled with a graphene-based Field Effect Transistor (FET)	Graphene-based	1.7 fM quantity of nucleic acid without the need for amplification within a short span of 15 min	Hajian et al. [58]
2	Graphene-based biosensing device functionalized with SARS-CoV-2 spike antibody (COVID-19 FET sensor)	Graphene-based device fabricated through 1-pyrenebutyric acid N-hydroxysuccinimide ester (PBASE)	Limit of detection (LOD) of 1 fg/mL	Seo et al. [59]
3	In-house built biosensor device (eCovSens)	Fluorine Doped Tin Oxide (FTO) electrode together with (AuNPs) and nCOVID-19 antibody	Could detect the nCOVID-19 antigen, ranging from 1 fM to 1 μM concentrations within 30–40 s	Mahari et al. [60]
4	Dual-functional, plasmonic biosensor Plasmonic Photothermal (PPT) and LSPR were also explored	2D gold nano-islands (AuNIs) functionalized with complementary DNA (cDNA) receptors and combining PPT effect and LSPR sensing technique	A high sensitivity towards the selected SARS-CoV-2 sequences, with a detection limit up to 0.22 pM conc	Qiu et al. [61]
5	Ploy amino ester carboxyl coated pcMNPs-based viral RNA extraction method for the sensitive detection of COVID-19	pcMNPs-RNA complexes directly introduced into Subsequent RT-PCR reactions and within 20 min identifying two different regions (ORFlab and N gene)	10-copy sensitivity and linear correlation between 10 and 10^5 Copies of SARS-CoV-2 pseudovirus particles	Zhao et al. [62]
6	Surface functionalised zinc ferrite NP's were fabricated successfully	Surface functionalised zinc ferrite NP's assisted potential RNA extraction protocol for active detection of COVID-19	Due to simple and cost-effective nature of this technique, it may provide a capable substitute for conventional techniques	Somvanshi et al. [63

NTS, long nucleic acid fragments have been sliced within fraction of time along with real-time processing of the output results is possible. In this technique, there is an internal panel where the amplification of SARS-CoV-2 unique genetic fragments occur and then the amplified fragments are sequenced with the help of an advanced nanopore platform [64]. The sequencing test is carried out on a MinION chip, and with the help of an indigenous bioinformatics station, the results are analysed

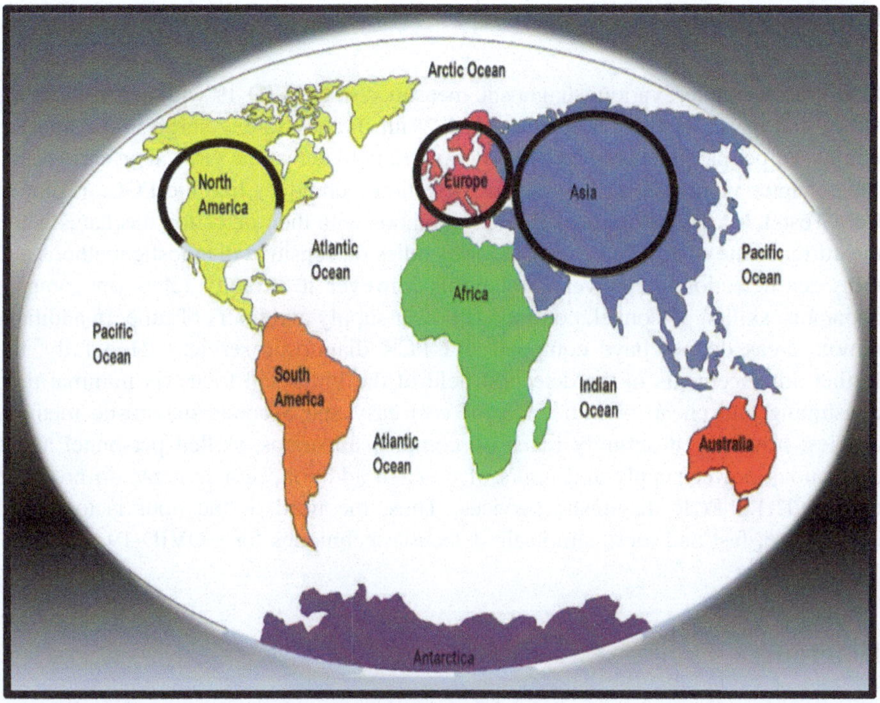

Fig. 7 Highest number of NTS-based testes conducted globally for COVID-19 infected people

continuously [65, 66]. Laboratories ranging from large to small scattered ones are using Oxford nanopore sequencing in order to sustain the sharing of genetic-sequencing data of coronavirus. Wang et al. reported simultaneous detection of SARS-CoV-2 along with other respiratory viruses via NTS method.

In a time span of 0–6 h, nearly 61 nucleic acid samples have been confirmed from potential suspected patients. NTS is a method which amplifies11 virulence-related and specific gene slices (orf1ab) of SARS-CoV-2 using a primer panel, and then the amplified fragments are sequenced on a nanopore platform followed [67]. Recently, IgG-IgM hybrid antibody colloidal Gold Method Tests reports have also been reported which claim rapid detection of recent COVID-19 infections [67]. In the global scenario, the highest use of MinION sequence NTS-based testes has been extended to highly affected countries around the world like USA, UK, France, New Zealand, Australia, Germany, Netherland, Spain and Korea. Figure 7 depicts highest number of NTS-based testes conducted globally for COVID-19 infected people.

6 Conclusion

In this book chapter, various diagnostic measures for COVID-19 with and without the aid of nanoparticles have been discussed. With the day-to-day surge in the affected number of people, it has become utterly important to detect the virus at an early stage. This chapter vividly describes various detection techniques like the POCs (Point of Care Tests), LAMP techniques, RTPCR methods with their detection mechanism and the current state of art. Detection platforms relies on sensitive diagnostic methods and tools for detection the novel coronavirus however it strongly relies on complex apparatus, skilled personnel, continuous power supply and hours of time. In addition, remote areas do not have equipped rRT-PCR diagnostic services. Hopefully, the further advancements in the detection field of the virus will focus on minimal time consuming and cheap or rather free of cost easy and accurate diagnostic methodologies; however, it strongly relies on complex apparatus, skilled personnel and a continuous power supply and hours of time. In addition, remote areas do not have equipped rRT-PCR diagnostic services. Thus, the need of the hour is to design easy-to-use, fast and more simplistic detection techniques for COVID-19.

References

1. Rabiee N, Bagherzadeh M, Ghasemi A, Zare H (2020) Point-of-Use rapid detection of SARS-CoV-2 : nanotechnology-enabled solutions for the COVID-19 pandemic
2. Nasrollahzadeh M, Sajjadi M, Soufi GJ, Iravani S, Varma RS (2020) Nanomaterials and nanotechnology-associated innovations against viral infections with a focus on coronaviruses. Nanomaterials 10(6):1–31. https://doi.org/10.3390/nano10061072
3. Nguyen T, Bang DD, Wolff A (2020) 2019 Novel coronavirus disease (COVID-19): paving the road for rapid detection and point-of-care diagnostics. Micromachines 11(3):1–7. https://doi.org/10.3390/MI11030306
4. Sivasankarapillai VS et al (2020) On facing the SARS-cov-2 (COVID-19) with combination of nanomaterials and medicine: Possible strategies and first challenges. Nanomaterials 10 (5):1–23. https://doi.org/10.3390/nano10050852
5. Weiss C et al (2020) Toward nanotechnology-enabled approaches against the COVID-19 pandemic. ACS Nano 14(6):6383–6406. https://doi.org/10.1021/acsnano.0c03697
6. Boopathi S, Poma AB, Kolandaivel P (2020) Novel 2019 coronavirus structure, mechanism of action, antiviral drug promises and rule out against its treatment. J Biomol Struct Dyn 1–14 https://doi.org/10.1080/07391102.2020.1758788
7. Thompson D, Lei Y (2020) Mini review: recent progress in RT-LAMP enabled COVID-19 detection. Sens Actuators Rep 100017 https://doi.org/10.1016/j.snr.2020.100017.
8. Statistics S (2020) Number of the coronavirus (COVID-19) cases across Indian states and union territories as of 13 July 2020, by type
9. Zhu X et al (2020) Multiplex reverse transcription loop-mediated isothermal amplification combined with nanoparticle-based lateral flow biosensor for the diagnosis of COVID-19. Biosens Bioelectron 166:112437https://doi.org/10.1016/j.bios.2020.112437
10. Li C, Zhao C, Bao J, Tang B, Wang Y, Gu B (2020) Laboratory diagnosis of coronavirus disease-2019 (COVID-19). Clin Chim Acta 510:35–46. https://doi.org/10.1016/j.cca.2020.06.045
11. Samson R, Navale GR, Dharne MS (2020) Biosensors: frontiers in rapid detection of COVID-19. 3 Biotech 10(9):1–9 https://doi.org/10.1007/s13205-020-02369-0.

12. Abdul W, Muhammad A, Atta Ullah K, Asmat A, Abdul B (2020) Role of nanotechnology in diagnosing and treating COVID-19 during the Pandemi. Int J Clin Virol 4(1):065–070 https://doi.org/10.29328/journal.ijcv.1001017.
13. Valdiglesias V, Laffon B (2020) The impact of nanotechnology in the current universal COVID-19 crisis. Let's not forget nanosafety!. Nanotoxicology 1–4 https://doi.org/10.1080/17435390.2020.1780332
14. Shen M et al (2020) Recent advances and perspectives of nucleic acid detection for coronavirus. J Pharm Anal 10(2):97–101. https://doi.org/10.1016/j.jpha.2020.02.010
15. Cheng VCC, Lau SKP, Woo PCY, Kwok YY (2007) Severe acute respiratory syndrome coronavirus as an agent of emerging and reemerging infection. Clin Microbiol Rev 20 (4):660–694. https://doi.org/10.1128/CMR.00023-07
16. Pooladanda V, Thatikonda S, Godugu C (2020) The current understanding and potential therapeutic options to combat COVID-19. Life Sci 254(May):117765 https://doi.org/10.1016/j.lfs.2020.117765
17. Somvanshi SB, Kharat PB, Saraf TS, Somwanshi SB, Shejul SB, Jadhav KM (2020) Multifunctional nano-magnetic particles assisted viral RNA-extraction protocol for potential detection of COVID-19. Mater Res Innov 00(00):1–6. https://doi.org/10.1080/14328917.2020.1769350
18. Use P et al (2020) SARS-CoV- 2(COVID-19) Fact Sheet
19. Goel S et al (2020) Resilient and agile engineering solutions to address societal challenges such as coronavirus pandemic. Mater Today Chem 17:100300https://doi.org/10.1016/j.mtchem.2020.100300
20. Tang Y, Schmitz JE, Persing DH, Stratton CW (2020) Crossm challenges. J Clin Microbiol 58(6):1–9
21. Kumar R, Nagpal S, Kaushik S, Mendiratta S (2020) COVID-19 diagnostic approaches: different roads to the same destination. VirusDisease 31(2):97–105. https://doi.org/10.1007/s13337-020-00599-7
22. Udugama B et al (2020) Diagnosing COVID-19: the disease and tools for detection. ACS Nano 14(4):3822–3835. https://doi.org/10.1021/acsnano.0c02624
23. Cevik M, Bamford CGG, Ho A (2020) COVID-19 pandemic—a focused review for clinicians. Clin Microbiol Infect 26(7):842–847. https://doi.org/10.1016/j.cmi.2020.04.023
24. Harapan H et al (2020) Coronavirus disease 2019 (COVID-19): a literature review. J Infect Public Health 13(5):667–673. https://doi.org/10.1016/j.jiph.2020.03.019
25. Yu Y et al (2020) Biosafety materials: an emerging new research direction of materials science from the COVID-19 outbreak. Mater Chem Front. https://doi.org/10.1039/d0qm00255k
26. Palmieri V, Papi M (2020) Can graphene take part in the fight against COVID-19?. Nano Today 33:100883https://doi.org/10.1016/j.nantod.2020.100883
27. Zhao Z, Cui H, Song W, Ru X, Zhou W, Yu X (2020) A simple magnetic nanoparticles-based viral RNA extraction method for efficient detection of SARS-CoV-2. 518055 https://doi.org/10.1101/2020.02.22.961268.
28. Mitchell SL, George KS (2020) Evaluation of the COVID19 ID NOW EUA assay. J Clin Virol 128(May):104429. https://doi.org/10.1016/j.jcv.2020.104429.
29. Dijkstra F, Van den Bossche T, Willekens B, Cras P, Crosiers D (2020) Myoclonus and Cerebellar Ataxia Following COVID-19. Mov Disord Clin Pract 7(8):974–976. https://doi.org/10.1002/mdc3.13049
30. Zhen W, Smith E, Manji R, Schron D, Berry GJ (2020) Clinical evaluation of three sample-to-answer platforms for detection of sars-cov-2. J Clin Microbiol 58(8):1–20. https://doi.org/10.1128/JCM.00783-20
31. Xiao M et al (2020) Multiple approaches for massively parallel sequencing of SARS-CoV-2 genomes directly from clinical samples. Genome Med 12(1):1–15. https://doi.org/10.1186/s13073-020-00751-4
32. Wang J et al (2020) Novel one-step single-tube nested quantitative real-time PCR assay for highly sensitive detection of SARS-CoV-2. Anal Chem 92(13):9399–9404. https://doi.org/10.1021/acs.analchem.0c01884

33. Suo T et al (2020) ddPCR: a more accurate tool for SARS-CoV-2 detection in low viral load specimens. Emerg Microbes Infect 9(1):1259–1268. https://doi.org/10.1080/22221751.2020.1772678
34. Zhang Y et al (2020) Rapid molecular detection of SARS-CoV-2 (COVID-19) Virus RNA using colorimetric LAMP. 2. https://doi.org/10.1101/2020.02.26.20028373
35. Moitra P et al (2020) Selective Naked-Eye detection of SARS-CoV-2 mediated by N Gene targeted antisense oligonucleotide capped plasmonic nanoparticles. ACS Nano 14(6):7617–7627. https://doi.org/10.1021/acsnano.0c03822
36. Visseaux B et al (2020) Evaluation of the qiastat-dx respiratory sars-cov-2 panel, the first rapid multiplex PCR commercial assay for sars-cov-2 detection. J Clin Microbiol 58(8) https://doi.org/10.1128/JCM.00630-20
37. Mujawar MA, Gohel H, Bhardwaj SK, Srinivasan S, Hickman N, Kaushik A (2020) Nano-enabled biosensing systems for intelligent healthcare: towards COVID-19 management. Mater Today Chem 17:100306https://doi.org/10.1016/j.mtchem.2020.100306
38. Adhikari S, Adhikari U, Mishra A, Guragain BS (2020) Nanomaterials for diagnostic, treatment and prevention of COVID-19. Appl Sci Technol Ann 1(1):155–164. https://doi.org/10.3126/asta.v1i1.30295
39. Statistics S (2020) Number of the coronavirus (COVID-19) cases across Indian states and union territories as of July 13, 2020
40. Thompson D, Lei Y (2020) Mini review: recent progress in RT-LAMP enabled COVID-19 detection. Sens Actuators Rep 100017 https://doi.org/10.1016/j.snr.2020.100017
41. Samson R, Navale GR, Dharne MS (2020) Biosensors: frontiers in rapid detection of COVID-19. 3 Biotech 10:1–9. https://doi.org/10.1007/s13205-020-02369-0
42. Zhu X, Wang X, Han L, et al (2020) Multiplex reverse transcription loop-mediated isothermal amplification combined with nanoparticle-based lateral flow biosensor for the diagnosis of COVID-19. Biosens Bioelectron 166:112437.https://doi.org/10.1016/j.bios.2020.112437
43. Li C, Zhao C, Bao J et al (2020) Laboratory diagnosis of coronavirus disease-2019 (COVID-19). Clin Chim Acta 510:35–46. https://doi.org/10.1016/j.cca.2020.06.045
44. Weiss C, Carriere M, Fusco L et al (2020) Toward nanotechnology-enabled approaches against the COVID-19 Pandemic. ACS Nano 14:6383–6406. https://doi.org/10.1021/acsnano.0c03697
45. Garg S, Kim L, Whitaker M et al (2019) Hospitalization rates and characteristics of patients hospitalized with laboratory-confirmed coronavirus disease 2019—COVID-NET, 14 States, March 1–30, 2020. MMWR Morb Mortal Wkly Rep 69(15):458–464. Available at: https://www.ncbi.nlm.nih.gov/pubmed/32298251.
46. Guan WJ, Ni ZY, Hu Y et al (2020) Clinical characteristics of coronavirus disease 2019 in China. N Engl J Med 82(18):1708–1720. Available at: https://www.ncbi.nlm.nih.gov/pubmed/32109013.
47. Wu C, Chen X, Cai Y et al (2020) Risk factors associated with acute respiratory distress syndrome and death in patients with coronavirus disease 2019 Pneumonia in Wuhan, China. JAMA Intern Med. Available at: https://www.ncbi.nlm.nih.gov/pubmed/32167524.
48. Palaiodimos L, Kokkinidis DG, Li W et al (39) Severe obesity, increasing age and male sex are independently associated with worse in-hospital outcomes, and higher in-hospital mortality, in a cohort of patients with COVID-19 in the Bronx, New York. Metabolism 108:154262. Available at: https://www.ncbi.nlm.nih.gov/pubmed/32422233.
49. Centers for Disease Control and Prevention (2020) Coronavirus disease 2019 (COVID-19): people who are at increased risk for severe illness. Available at: https://www.cdc.gov/coronavirus/2019-nco/need-extra-precautions/people-at-increased-risk.html. Accessed 26 June 2020
50. Lamb LE, Bartolone SN, Ward E, Chancellor MB (2020) Rapid detection of novel coronavirus (COVID19) by reverse transcription-loop-mediated isothermal amplification. SSRN Electron J. https://doi.org/10.2139/ssrn.3539654
51. Yu L, Wu S, Hao X et al (2020) Rapid colorimetric detection of COVID-19 coronavirus using a reverse transcriptional loop-mediated isothermal amplification (RT-LAMP) diagnostic platform: iLACO. Clin Chem. https://doi.org/10.1101/2020.02.20.20025874

52. Thompson D, Lei Y (2020) Mini review: recent progress in RT-LAMP enabled COVID-19 detection. Sens Actuators Rep 2(1):100017.https://doi.org/10.1016/j.snr.2020.100017
53. El-Tholoth M, Bau HH, Song J (2020) A single and two-stage, closed-tube, molecular test for the 2019 novel coronavirus (COVID-19) at home, clinic, and points of entry. ChemRxiv Prepr Serv Chemhttps://doi.org/10.26434/chemrxiv.11860137.
54. Broughton JP, Deng X, Yu G et al (2020) CRISPR–Cas12-based detection of SARS-CoV-2. Nat Biotechnol 38:870–874. https://doi.org/10.1038/s41587-020-0513-4
55. Joung J et al (2020) Point-of-care testing for COVID-19 using SHERLOCK diagnostics. medRxiv Prepr Serv Heal Sci. https://doi.org/10.1101/2020.05.04.20091231
56. Zhu X et al (2020) Multiplex reverse transcription loop-mediated isothermal amplification combined with nanoparticle-based lateral flow biosensor for the diagnosis of COVID-19. Biosens Bioelectron 166(May):112437 https://doi.org/10.1016/j.bios.2020.112437
57. Centers for Disease Control and Prevention (2020) Coronavirus disease 2019 (COVID-19): how to protect yourself & others. Available at: https://www.cdc.gov/coronavirus/2019-ncov/prevent-getting-sick/prevention-H.pdf. Accessed 7 July 2020
58. Yang T, Wang YC, Shen CF, Cheng CM (2020) Point-of-care RNA-based diagnostic device for Covid-19. Diagnostics 10(3):9–11. https://doi.org/10.3390/diagnostics10030165
59. Seo G et al (2020) Rapid detection of COVID-19 causative virus (SARS-CoV-2) in human nasopharyngeal swab specimens using field-effect transistor-based biosensor. ACS Nano 14 (4):5135–5142. https://doi.org/10.1021/acsnano.0c02823
60. Mahari S, Roberts A, Shahdeo D, Gandhi S (2020) eCovSens-ultrasensitive novel in-house built printed circuit board based electrochemical device for rapid detection of nCovid-19 antigen, a spike protein domain 1 of SARS-CoV-2. https://doi.org/10.1101/2020.04.24.059204.
61. Qiu G, Gai Z, Tao Y, Schmitt J, Kullak-Ublick GA, Wang J (2020) Dual-Functional Plasmonic Photothermal Biosensors for Highly Accurate Severe Acute Respiratory Syndrome Coronavirus 2 Detection. ACS Nano 14(5):5268–5277. https://doi.org/10.1021/acsnano.0c02439
62. Zhao Z, Cui H, Song W, Ru X, Zhou W, Yu X (2020) A simple magnetic nanoparticles-based viral RNA extraction method for efficient detection of SARS-CoV-2. 518055. https://doi.org/10.1101/2020.02.22.961268
63. Somvanshi SB, Kharat PB, Saraf TS, Somwanshi SB, Shejul SB, Jadhav KM (2020) Multifunctional nano-magnetic particles assisted viral RNA-extraction protocol for potential detection of COVID-19. Mater. Res Innov 1–6, 2020. https://doi.org/10.1080/14328917.2020.1769350
64. Pan Y, Zhang D, Yang P, Poon LLM, Wang Q (2020) Viral load of SARS-CoV-2 in clinical samples. Lancet Infect Dis 20(4):411–412. Available at: https://www.ncbi.nlm.nih.gov/pubmed/32105638
65. Rothe C, Schunk M, Sothmann P, et al. Transmission of 2019-nCoV infection from an asymptomatic contact in Germany. N Engl J Med. 2020;382(10):970–971. Available at: https://www.ncbi.nlm.nih.gov/pubmed/32003551.
66. Yu P, Zhu J, Zhang Z, Han Y, Huang L (2020) A familial cluster of infection associated with the 2019 novel coronavirus indicating potential person-to-person transmission during the incubation period. J Infect Dis 221(11):1757–1761. Available at: https://www.ncbi.nlm.nih.gov/pubmed/32067043.
67. Bai Y, Yao L, Wei T et al (2020) Presumed asymptomatic carrier transmission of COVID-19. JAMA 323(14):14061407. Availableat: https://www.ncbi.nlm.nih.gov/pubmed/32083643.
68. Tomás AL, de Almeida MP, Cardoso F et al (2019) Development of a gold nanoparticle-based lateral-flow Immunoassay for pneumocystis pneumonia serological diagnosis at point-of-care. Front Microbiol 10. https://doi.org/10.3389/fmicb.2019.02917

Chapter 7
Recent Developments Focusing Disinfectant Systems for Effective Inactivation of Coronaviruses

Arya Das, Mamata Mohapatra, and Suddhasatwa Basu

1 Introduction

The Covid-19 pandemic has been identified as a global public health emergency that has spread exponentially, affecting as many as 23 million people and with more than 8 lakh confirmed deaths up to August 26, 2020, leaving a colossal impact across 216 countries. The highly contagious coronavirus (also named SARS-CoV-2 by the International Committee on the Taxonomy of Viruses [ICTV]) is a matter of emergency global concern, with increasing fatalities and an absence of any established antiviral treatment or drug worsening the situation to a greater extent. With the foremost priority being the creation of a vaccine or antiviral drug the need of the hour focusses on proper practices of preventive measures and effective disinfection of public and private premises for limiting the transmission of the coronavirus. The SARS-CoV-2 infection is characterized by symptoms such as fever, cough, loss of taste and smell, respiratory disorders, etc., and can easily be transmitted from one person to another through aerosols, human contact, and surface contact. The World Health Organization (WHO) has already predicted a continuing lifespan for the coronavirus, recommending general day-to-day practices and anticipatory care as the only evidence-based means for the time being to restrict its spread. The slow resumption of different official and public activities requires the need for quick

A. Das (✉) · M. Mohapatra · S. Basu
CSIR-Institute of Minerals and Materials Technology, Bhubaneswar,
Odisha 751013, India
e-mail: mamata@immt.res.in

S. Basu
e-mail: sbasu@immt.res.in

A. Das
Academy of Scientific and Innovative Research (AcSIR), Ghaziabad,
Uttar Pradesh 201002, India

M. Mohapatra et al. (eds.), *COVID-19 Pandemic*, Materials Horizons:
From Nature to Nanomaterials, https://doi.org/10.1007/978-981-16-4372-9_7

disinfection at various public transport venues, commercial outlets, office spaces, and high-risk areas where the chances of transmission are high.

Many studies have focussed on the disinfection of coronaviruses for possible inactivation of the virus from both inanimate and animate surfaces. This chapter will provide a brief summary of the various disinfectants being used to combat Covid-19, further evaluating the efficacy of the different available disinfectants for possible intervention against the coronavirus.

1.1 Transmission and Longevity of Airborne Coronavirus

There have been concrete reports of pathogen transmission though aerosols contributing to the rapid airborne spread of respiratory transmission of the coronavirus, [1] such as fierce expiratory actions like sneezing and coughing [2]. The closest known virus strain SARS-CoV-1 was also reported to show transmission of virus-encapsulated aerosols from infected human carriers which could possibly result in high transmission among other persons [3]. There has not been any confirmatory report or sufficient evidence confirming the airborne transmission of Covid-19. The rapid spread of the coronavirus in the initial stages of virus confirmation urged researchers around the world to look into the possibility of airborne transmission. There have been diverse opinions: while some claim the transmission is limited to droplets within a short range of coughing and sneezing, there are assumptions predicting the rapid spread of the virus though minute particles (aerosols) from exhaled air to significant distances. Ordinary speech along with breathing is found to aerosolize a substantial number of respiratory particles, with louder vocals producing aerosols in higher magnitudes, ascertaining the risk of rapid transmission of the virus [4, 5]. Thus, there is an urgent need of proper investigation of the potency of aerosols to infect and transmit Covid-19 and there have already been some studies directed towards it. Lan et al. in a study collected air samples from multiple locations in Wuhan during the peak of the Covid-19 pandemic. The results reported infected aerosols from SARS-CoV-2 RNA found in and around Covid-19 hospitals and crowded departmental store entrances. Though the potential of aerosols to infect cells was not ascertained, the possibility exists that SARS-CoV-2 transmission may occur during breathing or talking, and could infect people up to considerable distances [6]. In contrast, a similar study by Ong et al. at Singapore did not find any infected SARS-CoV-2 aerosols in air samples of isolation centers treating Covid-19 patients, thus ruling out airborne transmission through aerosols, and instead designating the respiratory droplets of shorter range responsible for the same [7]. Another study by Santarpia et al. opposing Ong and group revealed viral RNA infection in two-third of air samples collected from an isolation facility treating critical Covid-19 patients in Nebraska [8]. A recent study by researchers using a nebulizer to produce artificial aerosols established the persistence time of the Covid-19 virus in aerosols to be up to three hours [9]. However, the WHO in its scientific brief has ruled out the possibility of airborne transmission based on lack of sufficient evidence. Responding to the research advancements carried out the WHO questions the uncertainty of virus transmission by its mere presence and the minimum dosage required to start the infection still remains unknown. The WHO also pointed out the study by van Doremalen and group to be highly artificial and lacking resemblance with normal human aerosol release conditions.

The definitions are confusing and the studies are scarce but the high risk of transmissibility still hovers around. The possible assumptions still remain adequate to take proper precautionary measures. One of the most common measures to follow is the mandatory wearing of face masks to contain the spread. Morawska et al. recommended adequate indoor ventilation with regular recirculation of air as one of the measures to reduce the risk of transmission in closed spaces [10]. Careful and proper circulation of air flow under negative pressure can be a measure for possible inhibition of the virus. The possibility of virus inhibition was presented in a study by Liu et al. that negative pressure ventilation and adequate air transfer levels within hospital rooms were effective in reducing infected SARS-CoV-2 aerosols [6, 11].

The likely transmission pathways and possible preventive measures have been elucidated figuratively in Fig. 1.

1.2 Transmission and Longevity of Coronavirus on Surfaces

SARS-CoV-2 can easily persist on infected surfaces through respiratory exhalations and can be transmitted to other people through surface contact. The persistence of the virus on various surfaces for considerable periods of time increases the risk of transmission to a greater extent. The coronavirus can be sustained on steel and copper surfaces from about four hours to four days, which can be extended up to nine days on plastic surfaces [12, 13]. Recent studies have established the longevity of the virus on different surfaces [12–15] and have been put together in a schematic

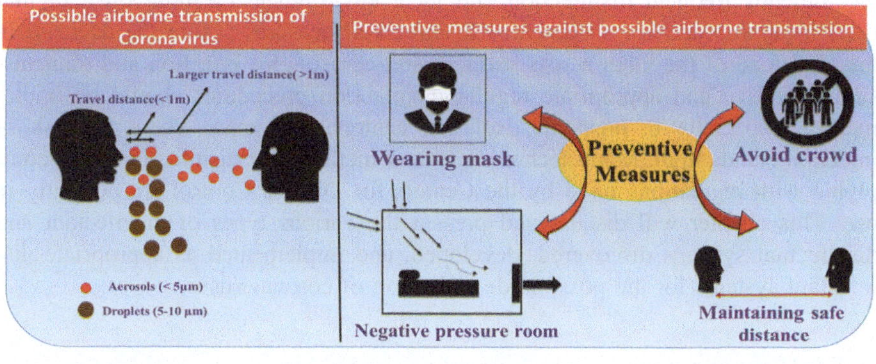

Fig. 1 Airborne transmission and preventive measures against SARS-CoV-2 airborne transmission

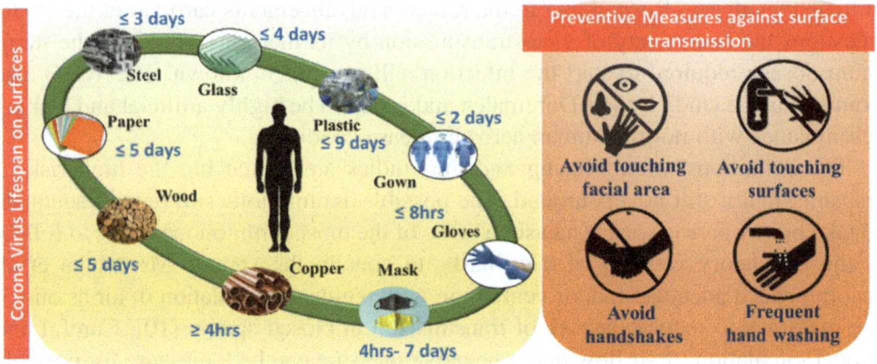

Fig. 2 The lifespan of coronaviruses on surfaces and preventive measures against surface exposure

view in Fig. 2. In a study Kampf et al. stated that the survival of human coronaviruses on plastic surfaces can be nine days, while veterinary coronavirus can persist for as long as 28 days. The report also inferred the lifetime of coronaviruses to be temperature dependent, with temperatures of around 30 degrees leading to shorter persistence of coronaviruses [13]. In another study Rajiv et al. studied the infection capability of coronavirus on various most-used day-to-day material surfaces, i.e., plastic, copper, stainless steel, and cardboard and revealed the high viral load capability of coronaviruses on these surfaces. The high infection capability was assisted with rapid linear decay of infection capability with time [16].

Although the dose of coronavirus on any surface and their potential to infect still stands unknown, the longevity of coronavirus on these surfaces can help in the rapid transmission of the virus. In this regard it very necessary to follow some basic human practices and preventive measures to reduce transmission, including frequent hand washing, avoiding contact with unknown surfaces, avoid touching the facial area, and handshakes.

Apart from the mandatory human practices mentioned above, the WHO also recommends frequent disinfection and local environment cleaning on a regular basis in appropriate ways. Repeated disinfection measures ensure the decrease in the viral load of the virus across surfaces and aerosols for infection and transmission. Effective and appropriate regular disinfection procedures should be implemented, especially in hospitals, isolation centers, and areas where the risk of infection stands high. Many technologies and methods for disinfection fully complying with regulations fixed by the Centers for Disease Control are currently in use. This chapter will discuss and present the various types of disinfectant and disinfectant systems discovered, developed, and implemented as appropriate disinfectant systems for the possible de-activation of coronaviruses.

2 Disinfectants Against Coronaviruses

Disinfection directs the use of chemicals to virtually decimate all acknowledged pathogenic microorganisms except those such as bacterial spores. Sterilization, on the other hand, kills all possible microorganism traits by deploying harsh physical and chemical conditions [17]. Cleaning, which usually refers to removing all the visible dust from the surface of animate and inanimate objects, when it is coupled with disinfection is termed sanitization. Cleaning is just a process of removing germs without killing them. Sanitizers, however, inactivate the microorganism load just like disinfectants, but disinfectants have broader kill claims. Disinfectants are mostly used for healthcare and household facilities, whereas sanitizers are mostly engaged in human disinfection use [18, 19]. A clear distinction has been provided in a schematic form in Fig. 3.

A disinfectant treats the microbes by terminating the cell structure, destroying their metabolism, and in turn inactivating them. A variety of disinfectants are already in use following the safety standards as recommended by the Centers for Disease Control and Prevention (CDC) and registered under the Food and Drug Administration agency (FDA) [20]. Disinfectants can broadly be categorized as physical or chemical disinfectants depending upon the technique of disinfection (Fig. 4).

SARS-CoV-2 being a large-enveloped virus (50–100 nm) can be disinfected easily compared to non-enveloped small viruses (<50 nm) [21]. However, among all the disinfectants that can be effectively used for the inactivation of Covid-19, no ideal disinfectant has yet been identified. It is also to be noted that unlike for chemical disinfectants, the Environmental Protection Agency (EPA) does not consistently review the safety or efficiency of physical disinfectants, thus does not endorse their efficiency against SARS-CoV-2. Accordingly, the EPA list consists only of surface disinfectants and not physical disinfecting devices. Disinfectants

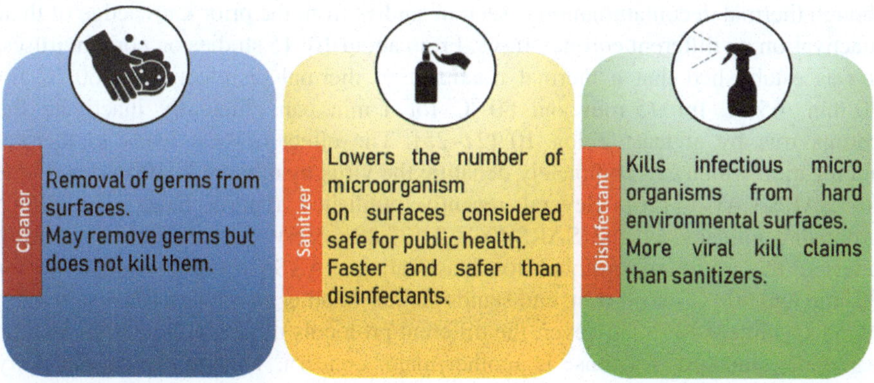

Fig. 3 The categorization of cleaner, sanitizer, and disinfectant for their appropriate employment for disinfection

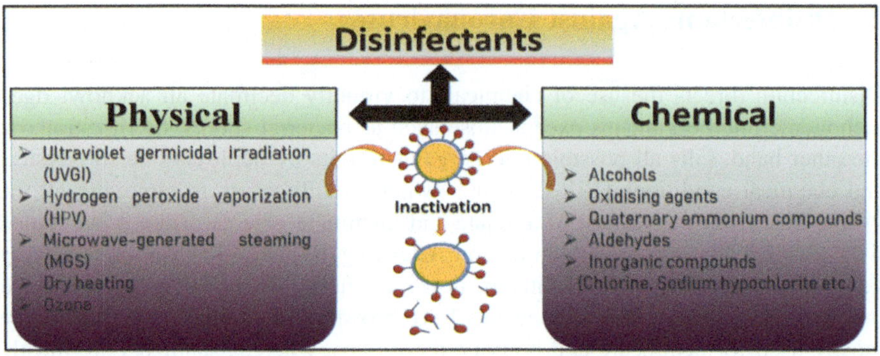

Fig. 4 The categorisation of physical and chemical disinfectants

have not only played a pivotal role for inactivating the coronavirus on different surfaces to stop their transmission, but have also largely contributed to the possible reuse of medical equipment and protective clothing, thus avoiding shortages in these items for frontline healthcare workers in this deadly pandemic. A brief discussion of the different disinfectants and their efficacy, along with their recommended safe use follows.

3 Physical Disinfectants

3.1 Dry Heating

The current global Covid-19 pandemic has resulted in the necessity of finding ways to address the possible shortages of hospital equipment and protective clothing and to develop procedures for their limited reuse. The efficiency of virus inactivation though thermal decontamination is seen in studies from the prior knowledge of their inactivation on different coronaviruses. From about 10–15 studies on coronaviruses, it was established that a thermal treatment of thermal disinfection at 60 °C for 30 min, 65 °C for 15 min and 80 °C for 1 min can efficiently inactivate the coronavirus by at least 4 log 10 [22–25]. The effect of heat leads to thermal aggregation which can completely denature the virus membrane in 10 min at 55 °C for SARS-CoV-1 [26]. Several recently published reports have also shown promising efficacy against SARS-CoV-2 [27,28]. Very recently Pastorino et al. inferred the optimum protocol for inactivating SARS-CoV-2 to be 56 °C for 30 min and 60 °C for 60 min, and stands similar to other enveloped RNA viruses in blood specimens [29]. However, the different protocols of decontamination and the parameter standards for reuse is another major concern. Though in one study dry heat was found to be more effective than chemical techniques considering the quality outcome of filtering face piece respirators (FFRs), temperatures above 100 °C have shown to degrade its performance [30,31]. Microwave heating has also found to degrade the overall usage quality, with their instant heat degrading the FFRs and making them unfit for reuse [32]. Thus, despite many optimistic results of different studies with other coronaviruses, the effective validation of the same for SARS-CoV-2 is still looked for in terms of standard protocols of usage, and adding to the reusable quality output considering the different types and qualities commercially available for large scale deployment.

3.2 *Microwave-Generated Steaming*

Microwave-generated steaming inactivation is an effective user-friendly mechanism employing microwaves to heat water sources, thus releasing steam to inactivate the pathogens across the surface by passing the released steam through it [33]. It is a realistic approach considering the easy availability and low cost of microwave ovens; it is, however, constrained by the absence of moisture [34]. Nevertheless, many studies have been carried out to prove the efficacy of microwave-based steaming systems and have pointed to some hopeful results. Heimbuch et al. established the inactivation by considerable 5-log of H1N1 influenza virus inoculated on FFRs within 2 min at 1250 watts without any significant mask degradation [34]. In another study Fisher et al. evaluated modified steam bags for decontamination of FFRs with encouraging results of >3 log inactivation within 90 s at 1100 watts without any effect on the filtration efficiency of FFRs even after three cycles [35]. Lore et al. similarly observed extra dose removal of A/H5N1 virus by >4 log without any significant effect on the filtering performance of FFRs [33].

All these studies seem to be encouraging, however there have been no real studies on SARS-CoV-2 until now. Additionally, the homogeneity of steam penetration for uniform decontamination and the limitation of moisture absence along with the scale of decontamination still needs to be addressed for benchmarking the process.

3.3 *Ozone*

Activated oxygen—also known as ozone—is a powerful oxidizing agent that is proposed to be an effective safe and efficient inactivating agent, without tampering the surfaces, given that they operate at room temperatures, unlike techniques which use harmful UV rays, severe chemicals, or heat. Ozone gas, which has a higher density than air, is already reported to be effective against various types of viruses suspended in air, on surfaces, or in water [36, 37]. Ozone was reported to be highly effective with wide deployment for environment purification during the SARS-Cov-1 pandemic. Studies revealed the inactivation potential of ozone against enveloped viruses by destroying the outer lipid membrane of viral RNA via oxidation. There are no studies on its efficacy against SARS-CoV-2, however, a very recent study by Lee et al. on HCoV-229E human virus (considered to be the surrogate of SARS-CoV-2), established the ability of ozone to inactivate HCoV-229E within 1 min of ozone exposure. The ozone gas produced by a plasma generator showed null degradation in the structural properties of the face masks investigated even after excessive repeated ozone gas exposures [38].

Though the efficacy of ozone against SARS-CoV-2 is too immature to assume, given its easy and inexpensive production and rapid inactivation potential ozone gas can go a long way in the fight against the Covid-19 pandemic.

3.4 Hydrogen Peroxide Vaporization

Vaporized hydrogen peroxide is a well-established decontamination technique widely adapted in hospitals owing to its high efficacy against surface pathogens. The vaporization of the hydrogen peroxide oxidizing agent is considered to be a practical and cost-effective contamination method employing vapors to denature viruses [39, 40]. The decontamination is carried out with varying H_2O_2 concentrations depending upon the method: 30–35% for vapor; and 5–6% for aerosol-based decontamination [41]. Tuladhar et al. proved the efficacy of vaporized hydrogen peroxide against respiratory viruses across different surfaces with results of >4 log reduction for poliovirus on stainless steel and wood panels, whereas >3 and >3.5 log reduction was achieved for the influenza virus on steel surfaces and wood panels respectively [42].

Apart from being employed as an effective decontamination technology in hospitals for surface and room sterilization, the H_2O_2 vaporization technique has also gained ample attention as an effective option for mask decontamination for their possible reuse. The Dutch National Institute for Public Health and Environment (RIVM) reported successful quality retrieval of FFP2 face masks earlier subjected to inactivation after two cycles of low pressure 3 M H_2O_2 decontamination [43]. Swatch et al. reported decontamination of 100 N95 masks with 6 log reduction (Geobacillus stearothermophilus spores indiactor) using 35% H_2O_2 with a 45 min standard operation time of one cycle. The functional and structural stability were commendable even after 50 cycles; a reuse cycle of 30 times was recommended [44]. Similar decontamination efficacy was also corroborated by another study in Battelle Memorial Institute, Ohio. The Battelle Decontamination System was developed that reflected parallel efficiency and nominal structural misfits even after 50 cycles when FFRs were subjected to a gassing time of 20 min in a dwell time of 150 min [45]. There are presently no concrete studies or conclusive evidence on the efficacy of H_2O_2 on decontamination of SARS-CoV-2. One recent study, however, denies that there is sufficient proof, and recommends additional treatment with ethanol till further tangible evidence is available [46].

Hydrogen peroxide vaporization can serve as a safe and environmentally friendly practice for being accepted as a sustainable future decontamination technique. However, some major concerns on the lack of evidence for effective use of H_2O_2 against SARS-CoV-2, the toxicity of residual H_2O_2, and off-gassing from the inner layers of respirators all still need to be addressed.

3.5 Ultraviolet Germicidal Irradiation

Radiation inactivation has long been known as an effective decontamination technique having the potential for a wide range of disinfections upon surfaces, liquids, and air [47]. Among all the spectral ranges of UV, UV-C with a wavelength around 254 nm, closest to the bacterial killing wavelength of 264 nm has been employed widely to inactivate viral load across surfaces [48–50].

The germicidal efficacy of UV-C corresponds to damage of DNA and RNA via absorbing photons of higher energy, resulting in pyrimidine by-products, which constrains the microbes to replicate, thus inactivating them [51]. Mercury lamps that were often employed for UV-C generation and widely used in air and water purifiers were recently banned by the United Nations for export and import, and replaced with LED lamps owing to the concern of mercury pollution [52]. The mercury lamps further emitted an ozone that was toxic to humans as a by-product, though the emitted ozone was considered to be an efficacy enhancer owing to its self-inactivating properties [53]. However, the UV-LED lamp sources have also delivered equivalent results [54].

Ultraviolet Germicidal Irradiation (UVGI) technology has been well established and employed for public health interventions, due to its efficiency against all bacteria and viruses. Lin et al. in one study elucidated the efficacy of UV-C to be higher than its counterparts UV-A and ethanol [55]. UV-C inactivation has also been highly efficient in combating SARS-CoV-1 and MERS-CoV [56]. The most essential parameter of UV disinfection lies in the dosage of UV-C used. In one study an UV dose of 1 J cm^{-2} for 60–70 s led to >3 log reduction of H1N1 infected FFRs. The dosage was also supported by subsequent studies, and it was reported that a dosage higher than J cm^{-2} led to a decrease in efficacy of inactivation [57, 58]. The optimum dosage of inactivation is found to be a variable of the surface posture along with the susceptible species involved. To support the claim in one study Tseng et al. claimed the UV dosage for double-stranded DNA and viruses was doubled compared to single-stranded DNA and viruses to achieve 90% inactivation. The dosage is also found to vary with moisture content, provided the moisture content alters the efficacy of dosage inactivation making it more resistant to UV [59, 60].

The prevailing pandemic has led to a rapid development of various UV-based technologies for possible inactivation of coronaviruses. In one such development Orbit from Michigan have developed a mask sanitizer-based UV device [61]. A group at Binghamton University assembled large UV bulbs for the possible

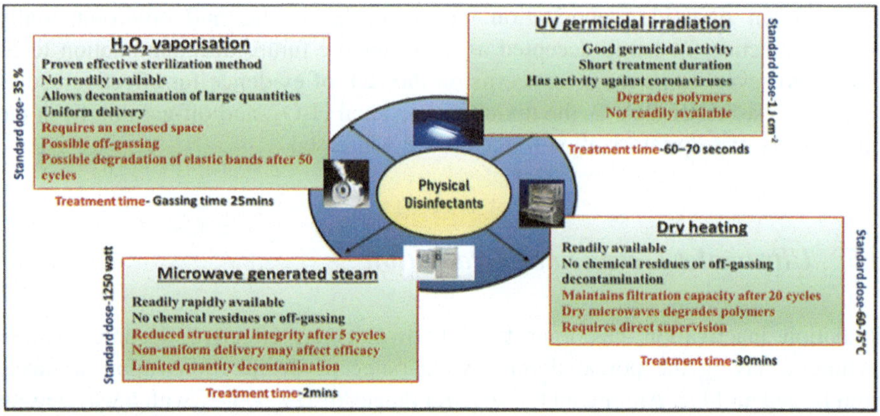

Fig. 5 The different physical disinfectants with their appropriate usage and efficacy

sterilization of coronaviruses. The station assembled worked on a computational model based on previous dosage information of UV against SARS and other coronaviruses [62]. Similarly, researchers at Nebraska Medicine used UV towers diagonally placed to possibly inactivate SARS-CoV-2 infection of N95 masks placed between them [63]. ACRI of India successfully developed UV disinfection trolleys that were operational with a speed of 5ft/minute, and that can cover rooms as large as 400 sq. ft. with an efficacy of 99% inactivation in 30 min [64].

The established potential of highly efficient inactivation through UV, however, should mandatorily be assisted by validated dosimetry. The inappropriate dosage of inadequate inactivation may possess a serious threat to health workers. The UV inactivation should assess the proper reach to the shadowed areas of different surfaces. Furthermore, UV is also reported to degrade polymers [61], which also mandates the consideration of the treated FFRs for reuse subject to degradation. The adverse effect of human health upon exposure to UV should also be deliberated, to recommend standard protocols of use.

A graphic representation of all the physical disinfectants with their appropriate usage and efficacy has been presented in Fig. 5.

4 Chemical Disinfectants

A large number of chemical disinfectants have been introduced into the healthcare setting which include chlorine and chlorine compounds (bleach), alcohols, glutaraldehyde, formaldehyde, hydrogen peroxide, phenolics, peracetic acid, iodophors, and quaternary ammonium compounds (Quats). Commercialized products in markets using these chemical compounds for COVID-19 are considered to be unique, and should have prior registration with the Environmental Protection

Agency (EPA), or should have been cleared by the Food and Drug Administration agency (FDA) [65]. Several viruses have been recognized in their ranking for tolerance to chemical disinfectants by Centers for Disease Control and prevention (CDCs). On this basis, viruses are categorized as enveloped viruses, large non-enveloped viruses (in the range of 50–100 nm), and small non-enveloped viruses (<50 nm). Wherein, the order of inactivation was found to be: enveloped > large-enveloped > small-enveloped. Hence rhinovirus, which is a small-enveloped virus, is hard to inactivate in comparison to enveloped viruses, i.e., SARS-CoV-2, which can be easily inactivated with the use of the aforementioned disinfectants [21]. There are a wide range of disinfectants introduced by the EPA but there is no ideal disinfectant at present. The entire range of chemical disinfectants is composed of manmade or natural surfactants, oil, and soap. The majority of market products used as disinfectants contain quaternary ammonium as an active ingredients (Quats). Some other market products may include mixtures of ethanol, isopropanol, triethylene glycol, peroxyacetic acid, glycolic acid, octanoic acid, hydrogen peroxide, sodium hypochlorite, and L-lactic acid [66]. Below are listed the most frequently used disinfectants with their effects on microbes, bacteria, and viruses.

4.1 Chlorine and its Derivatives

Generally, free chlorine is used as a disinfectant due to its ability to immediately penetrate the lipid membrane of microbes to react with the proteins present in the polymerase complex and nucleocapsid [67]. Whereas in the case of the Covid-19 enveloped virus, free chlorine leads to the loss of its ability to bind with the host receptor. First, free chlorine damages the viral capsids allowing free chlorine to interact with viral RNA and then further to damage its viral genomes which causes loss of binding [68]. Use of chlorine can be carried out in gas form (chlorine dioxide—ClO_2) or liquid form (hypochlorite). Chlorine dioxide is a more powerful oxidant than hypochlorite.

Chlorine dioxide was found to be a powerful disinfectant with strong inhibitory effects on parasites and microbes. Even in vitro usage, chlorine dioxide has shown a capability to potently supress porcine reproductive and respiratory syndrome [69]. It has also been employed in irrigation water to prevent the formation of organ halogens as by-products [70]. The other chlorinated disinfectant is NaOCl (sodium hypochlorite) which has an effective antimicrobial activity with a broad range of microbe killing. Moreover, treating water containing levels of amino acids or peptides with chlorinated disinfectants can pose risks to human health. Organic nitrogen compounds present in water can react with chlorine to form organo-chloramines which are toxic by nature. Further, if chlorine reacts with peptides, then chlorinated compounds of peptides are relatively more stable than chlorinated amine compounds [71].

4.2 Alcohols

Several alcohols can be used as disinfectants, such as ethanol and isopropyl alcohol both at a concentration of 70%. Ethanol is generally used in hand-hygiene products in the form of hand rubs, foam, or gels, and the WHO has also recommended ethanol in the 80% (v/v) range as an essential medicine categorized in alcohol-based hand rubs. Ethanol was found to be useful in dealing with the transmissible gastroenteritis virus (TGEV), which was reduced in the suspension test of 5 min with the use of 4.5 log 10 ethanol [72]. Coronaviruses such as the Middle East Respiratory Syndrome (MERS) and Severe Acute Respiratory Syndrome (SARS) can become inactivated with the usage of 70% ethanol and 1% NaOCl. Similarly, it is believed that Covid-19 will be affected likewise [13].

4.3 Quaternary Ammonium (Quats)

One other type of disinfectant are quaternary ammonium (Quats) cations, which have antimicrobial and spermicidal activity, and can inactivate the encapsulated viruses or enveloped viruses having long alkyl chains [73]. Quaternary ammonium has showed the potential of inactivating avian influenza from plastic and steel carriers after exposure of just 60 min [74]. Some of the examples of quaternary ammonium are methylbenzethonium chloride, benzalkonium chloride, benzethonium chloride, cetylpyridinium chloride, cetrimonium, cetrimide, tetraethylammonium bromide, cetalconium chloride, didecyldimethylammonium chloride, and domiphene bromide. Quats are positively charged ions, and if the surfaces are not thoroughly rinsed before the application of quaternary ammonium and anions are not totally removed, then the Quats may electrically neutralize with the anions and its antimicrobial action can be totally inactivated in that case. Moreover, residue of complex detergent Quats can easily provide the nutrients for the growth of microbes and bacteria. If they are left uncleaned, then they may colonize and form biofilm. These biofilms thrive in environmental conditions that have moisture and soil in contact with the surfaces, particularly for locker rooms, food service areas, restrooms, and similar places [66].

4.4 Oxidizing Agents

Peroxide-based oxidizing agents such as hydrogen peroxide and peroxyacetic acid have found to be highly efficient disinfectants for microbe inactivation. Both compounds release hydroxyl radicals oxidizing thiol and disulphide bonds of the outer lipid membranes to denature them [75–77]. The virucidal efficiency of hydrogen peroxide is well established by its potency in the de-activation of

SARS-CoV-1 within one minute at very low concentrations of <3% [78]. Peroxyacetic acid, on the other hand, is reported to be more effective against a broad range of pathogens at even lower concentrations than peroxide, thus being widely used to disinfect hospital spaces and medical devices [75, 79].

4.5 Formaldehyde and Glutaraldehyde

Formaldehyde and glutaraldehyde can readily disinfect susceptible targets by alkylating the outer membrane and rupturing the lipid membrane to denature them and rendering them inactivated for possible replication. Both the aldehydes have already proved effective against coronaviruses at concentrations as low as 0.3–3% within 2 min [80, 81]. However, formaldehyde is constrained in its usage, as it is a carcinogenic aldehyde assisted with strong odour and fumes [75, 79].

4.6 Serious Health Risks with Frequent Use of Disinfectants

As Covid-19 increases rapidly around the globe, it gives rise to anxiety and panic in every individual in terms of catching the infection. This allows for the frequent and increased use of chemical disinfectants which might lead to secondary disasters in our ecosystems and human health. Extensive research has been carried out on the effects of frequent exposure to chemical disinfectants. Frequently used disinfectants such as chlorine and chlorine derivative, Quats, and alcohols are linked to increased risk of COPD (Chronic Obstructive Pulmonary Disease), eye irritation, and asthma when used very frequently [66, 82]. The residue of chemicals on the surfaces can be inhaled and airborne-transmitted, which can lead to poor air quality and allergic or asthmatic reactions in sensitive people. These chemical disinfectant residues can cause impairment of the central nervous system, eye and skin irritation, oxidative damage, reproductive disorders, respiratory issues including occupational asthma, cancer, and other human health risks [83]. Moreover, Quats can possibly cause fertility problems in the female and male reproduction processes. Due to the circulation of some misleading information on social media for Covid-19, individuals can get panicky, anxious, and fearful, which leads to extreme actions. It has been reported that people have even washed fruits and vegetables with disinfectants, applied them to skin, and also ingested them [84]. These actions could be very dangerous and could cause human health risks in terms of permanent damage to the nervous system, coma, seizures, blindness, or death. Further, bleach solutions like NaOCl can be very harsh on the skin and can result in irritation in several parts of body including the eyes and skin [85]. Moreover, bleach ingestion can give rise to hyperchloremia, lung injury, ARDS, hypernatremia, and hyperchloremia. In addition, chlorine bleach exposure can result in gastrointestinal irritation, asthma symptoms, ear, nose, and throat lesions and mucosal erosions [86]. Some of the

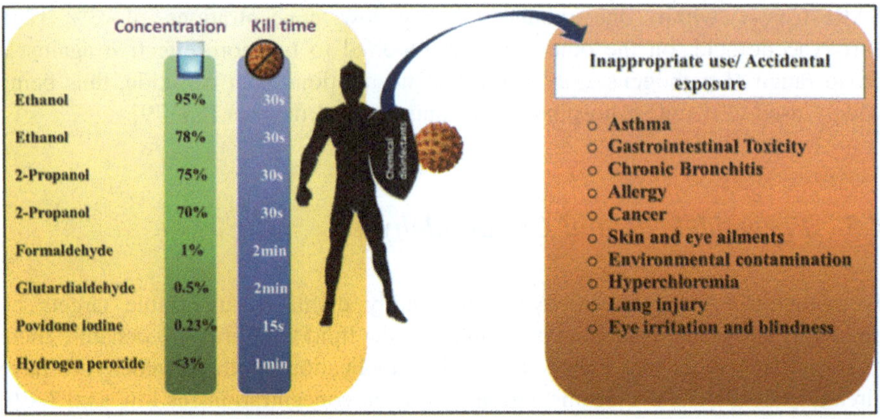

Fig. 6 The different available chemical disinfectants with their dosage and kill time along with possible health hazards accompanying inappropriate use

cleaning products which contain caustic materials can, if accidentally ingested, cause gastrointestinal toxicity [87].

A schematic of all the adopted chemical disinfectants, their dosage along with accompanying health hazards has been presented in Fig. 6.

5 Conclusion

The ongoing Covid-19 pandemic has become an urgent public health concern with an exponential rise in the number of cases and fatality rates, without any possibility of a vaccine in the near future. Meanwhile, although there are many disinfectants available for possible interventions against SARS-CoV-2, nevertheless, the efficacy of individual disinfectants within each system with their appropriate usage is highly recommended. Human exposure to various disinfectants should be minimized, with appropriate dosages and methods of operation carried out, to avoid any additional possible human health hazards. All the recommended preventive measures such as social distancing, wearing face masks, regular hand hygiene, and respiratory practices should be strictly followed, coupled with regular disinfection of potential susceptible risk areas. Practicing individual hygiene measures, along with proper disinfection methods, still shines as a ray of hope against combating Covid-19 until any drug or vaccine arrives.

References

1. Tellier R, Li Y, Cowling BJ, Tang JW (2019) Recognition of aerosol transmission of infectious agents: a commentary. BMC Infect Dis 19(1):101. https://doi.org/10.1186/s12879-019-3707-y
2. Bourouiba L, Dehandschoewercker E, Bush JWM (2014) Violent expiratory events: On coughing and sneezing. J Fluid Mech 745:537–563. https://doi.org/10.1017/jfm.2014.88
3. Jayaweera M, Perera H, Gunawardana B, Manatunge J (2020) Transmission of Covid-19 virus by droplets and aerosols: a critical review on the unresolved dichotomy. Environ Res 109819
4. Morawska L, Johnson GR, Ristovski ZD, Hargreaves M, Mengersen K, Corbett S, Chao CYH, Li Y, Katoshevski D (2009) Size distribution and sites of origin of droplets expelled from the human respiratory tract during expiratory activities. J Aerosol Sci 40(3): 256–269. https://doi.org/10.1016/j.jaerosci.2008.11.002
5. Asadi S, Wexler AS, Cappa CD, Barreda S, Bouvier NM, Ristenpart WD (2019) Aerosol emission and superemission during human speech increase with voice loudness. Sci Rep 9(1): 2348. https://doi.org/10.1038/s41598-019-38808-z
6. Liu Y et al (2020) Aerodynamic characteristics and RNA concentration of SARS-CoV-2 aerosol in Wuhan hospitals during Covid-19 outbreak. BioRxiv
7. Ong SWX et al (2020) Air, surface environmental, and personal protective equipment contamination by severe acute respiratory syndrome coronavirus 2 (SARS-CoV-2) from a symptomatic patient. Jama 323(16):1610–1612
8. Santarpia JL et al (2020) Aerosol and surface transmission potential of SARS-CoV-2. medRxiv
9. Van Doremalen N et al (2020) Aerosol and surface stability of SARS-CoV-2 as compared with SARS-CoV-1. New England J Med 382(16):1564–1567
10. Morawska L, Junji C (2020) Airborne transmission of SARS-CoV-2: the world should face the reality. Environ Int 105730
11. Khalil EE (2005) Air-conditioning systems' developments in hospitals: comfort, air quality, and energy utilization. Proc Clima Med 85
12. Moriyama M, Hugentobler WJ, Iwasaki A (2020) Seasonality of respiratory viral infections. Ann Rev Virol 7 https://doi.org/10.1146/annurev-virology-012420-022445. PMID 32196426
13. Kampf G, Todt D, Pfaender S, Steinmann E (2020) Persistence of coronaviruses on inanimate surfaces and its inactivation with biocidal agents. J Hospit Infect. In press
14. Yu IT, Qiu H, Tse LA, Wong TW (2014) Severe acute respiratory syndrome beyond Amoy Gardens: completing the incomplete legacy. Clin Infect Dis 58:683–686
15. Van Doremalen N, Bushmaker T, Morris DH et al (2020) Aerosol and surface stability of SARS-CoV-2 as compared with SARS-CoV-1. New Eng J Med 17 (Online ahead of print)
16. Suman R, Javaid M, Haleem A, Vaishya R, Bahl S, Nandan D (2020) Sustainability of coronavirus on different surfaces. J Clin Exp Hepatol
17. Division of Oral Health—Infection Control Glossary. U.S. Centers for Disease Control and Prevention. Archived from the Original on 13 Apr 2016. Retrieved 9 Apr 2019
18. Cleaning. Food Standards Agency. Retrieved 9 Apr 2020, Mid Sussex District Council, UK
19. Green Cleaning, Sanitizing, and Disinfecting: A Curriculum for Early Care and Education (PDF). Retrieved 9 April 2019
20. Disinfection & Sterilization Guidelines. Guidelines Library: Infection Control. CDC. In: Archived from the original on 12 Jan 2018. 28 Dec 2016. Retrieved 12 January 2018
21. Cascella M, Rajnik M, Cuomo A, Dulebohn SC, Di Napoli R (2020) Features, evaluation and treatment of coronavirus (Covid-19). Treasure Island (FL): StatPearls
22.] Rabenau HF, Cinatl J, Morgenstern B, Bauer G, Preiser W, Doerr HW (2005) Stability and inactivation of SARS coronavirus. Med Microbiol Immunol 194:1e6
23. Darnell ME, Taylor DR (2006) Evaluation of inactivation methods for severe acute respiratory syndrome coronavirus in noncellular blood products. Transfusion 46:1770e7

24. Yunoki M, Urayama T, Yamamoto I, Abe S, Ikuta K (2004) Heat sensitivity of a SARS-associated coronavirus introduced into plasma products. Vox Sanguinis 87:302e3
25. Saknimit M, Inatsuki I, Sugiyama Y, Yagami K. Virucidal efficacy of physico-chemical treatments against coronaviruses and parvoviruses of laboratory animals. Jikken Dobutsu Exp Animals 37:341e5
26. Wang Y, Wu X, Wang Y, Li B, Zhou H, Yuan G et al (2004) Low stability of nucleocapsid protein in SARS virus. Biochemistry 43:11103e8
27. Fischer R, Morris DH, van Doremalen N, Sarchette S, Matson J, Bushmaker T et al (2020) Assessment of N95 respirator decontamination and re-use for SARS-CoV-2. medRxiv, [Pre-Print]. https://doi.org/10.1101/2020.04.11.20062018
28. Kumar A, Kasloff SB, Leung A, Cutts T, Strong JE, Hills K et al (2020) N95 Mask decontamination using standard hospital sterilization technologies. medRxiv, [Pre-Print]. https://doi.org/10.1101/2020.04.05.20049346
29. Boris P, Franck T1, Magali G1, de Xavier L, Remi NC (2020) Evaluation of heating and chemical protocols for inactivating SARS-CoV-2.Viruses 12(7):735
30. Heimbuch BK, Wallace WH, Kinney K, Lumley AE, Wu CY, Woo MH, Wander JD (2011) Am J Infect Control 39:e1–e9
31. Lin TH, Chen CC, Huang SH, Kuo CW, Lai CY, Lin WY (2017) PLoS One 12:e0186217
32. Viscusi DJ, Bergman MS, Eimer BC, Shaffer RE (2009) Ann Occup Hyg 53:815–827
33. Lore MB, Heimbuch BK, Brown TL, Wander JD, Hinrichs SH (2012) Ann Occup Hyg 56:92–101
34. Heimbuch BK, Wallace WH, Kinney K, Lumley AE, Wu CY, Woo MH, Wander JD (2011) Am J Infect Control 39:e1–e9
35. Fisher EM, Williams JL, Shaffer RE (2011) PLoS One 6:e18585
36. Hudson JB, Sharma M, Vimalanathan S (2009) Development of a practical method for using ozone gas as a virus decontaminating agent. Ozone Sci Eng 31(3):216–223. https://doi.org/10.1080/01919510902747969
37. Mastanaiah N, Johnson JA, Roy S (2013) Effect of dielectric and liquid on plasma sterilization using dielectric barrier discharge plasma. PLoS One. 8(8):e70840 312. https://doi.org/10.1371/journal.pone.0070840
38. Lee J, Bong C, Bae PK, Abafog AT, Baek SH, Shin YB, Bak MS, Park S (2020) Fast and easy disinfection of coronavirus-contaminated face masks using ozone gas produced by a dielectric barrier discharge plasma generator. medRxiv
39. Zonta W, Mauroy A, Farnir F, Thiry E (2016) Virucidal Efficacy of a hydrogen peroxide nebulization against murine norovirus and feline calicivirus, Two surrogates of human norovirus. Food Environ Virol 8:275–282. https://doi.org/10.1007/s12560-016-9253-5
40. Fraise A, Maillard JY, Sattar S (2013) Russell, 5th edn. Hugo & Ayliffe's principles and practice of disinfection, Preservation and Sterilization, Wiley-Blackwell, United Kingdom
41. Weber DJ, Kanamori H, Rutala WA (2016) Curr Opin Infect Dis 29:424–431
42. Tuladhar E, Terpstra P, Koopmans M, Duizer E (2012) J Hosp Infect 80:110–115
43. Dutch National Institute for Public Health and the Environment (RIVM) (2020) Reuse of FFP2 masks 1–5
44. Schwartz A, Stiegel M, Greeson N, Vogel A, Thomann W, Brown M, Sempowski GD, Alderman TS, Condreay JP, Burch J, Wolfe C, Smith B, Lewis S (2020) Appl. Biosaf. 25:67–70
45. Battelle CCDS Critical Care Decontamination System. https://www.battelle.org/docs/default-source/commercialofferings/industrysolutions/732_battelle-critical-care-deconsystem_technical-summaryf.pdf. Accessed Apr 2020
46. Ludwig-Begall LF, Wielick C, Dams L, Nauwynck H, Demeuldre PF, Napp A, Thiry E (2020) The use of germicidal ultraviolet light, vaporized hydrogen peroxide and dry heat to decontaminate face masks and filtering respirators contaminated with a SARS-CoV-2 surrogate virus. J Hosp Infect
47. Reed NG (2010) Public Health Rep 125:15–27
48. Casini B, Tuvo B, Cristina ML, Spagnolo AM, Totaro M, Baggiani A, Privitera GP (2019) Int J Environ Res Public Health 16:1–10

49. Guridi A, Sevillano E, de la Fuente I, Mateo E, Eraso E, Quindos G (2019) Int J Environ Res Public Health 16:1–11
50. Yang JH, Wu UI, Tai HM, Sheng WH, Microbiol J (2019) Immunol Infect 52:487–493
51. Kowalski W (2010) Ultraviolet germicidal irradiation handbook: UVGI for air and surface disinfection. Springer science & business media
52. Kim DK, Kang DH (2018) Appl Environ Microbiol 84:1–11
53. Kim J, Jang J (2018) Aerosol Sci Technol 52:557–566
54. Nunayon SS, Zhang H, Lai ACK (2020) Indoor Air 30:180–191
55. Lin TH, Tang FC, Hung PC, Hua ZC, Lai CY (2018) Indoor Air 28:754–762
56. Bedell K, Buchaklian AH, Perlman S (2016) Infect Control Hosp Epidemiol 37:598–599
57. Mills D, Harnish DA, Lawrence C, Sandoval-Powers M, Heimbuch BK (2018) Am J Infect Control 46:e49–e55
58. Fisher EM, Shaffer RE (2011) J Appl Microbiol 110:287–295
59. Memarzadeh F, Olmsted RN, Bartley JM (2010) Am J Infect Control 38:S13–S24
60. Tseng CC, Li CS (2007) J Occup Environ Hyg 4:400–405
61. Hamzavi IH, Lyons AB, Kohli I, Narla S, Parks-Miller A, Gelfand JM, Lim HW, Ozog D (2020) J Am Acad Dermatol https://doi.org/10.1016/j.jaad.2020.03.085
62. Bauchner H, Fontanarosa PB, Livingston EH (2020) Conserving supply of personal protective equipment—a call for ideas. JAMA 323(19):1911–1911
63. Lowe JJ et al (2020) N95 filtering facemask respirator ultraviolet germicidal irradiation (uvgi) process for decontamination and reuse. Tech Rep Nebraska Med
64. Sarada BV, Vijay R, Johnson R, Rao TN, Padmanabham G (2020) Fight against COVID-19: ARCI's technologies for disinfection. Trans Indian Nat Acad Eng 5(2):349–354
65. Rutala WA, Weber DJ (2008) Guideline for disinfection and sterilization in healthcare facilities
66. Rai NK, Ashok A, Akondi BR (2020) Consequences of chemical impact of disinfectants: safe preventive measures against Covid-19. Crit Rev Toxicol 1–8
67. Ye Y, Wigginton K (2018) Enveloped virus inactivation by UV and chlorine disinfection. Presented at the Abstracts of Papers of the American Chemical Society, Amer Chemical SOC 1155 16TH ST, NW, Washington, DC 20036 USA
68. Fuzawa M, Araud E, Li J, Shisler JL, Nguyen TH (2019) Free chlorine disinfection mechanisms of rotaviruses and human norovirus surrogate Tulane virus attached to fresh produce surfaces. Environ Sci Technol 53:11999–12006
69. Zhu Z, Guo Y, Yu P, Wang X, Zhang X, Dong W, Liu X, Guo C (2019) Chlorine dioxide inhibits the replication of porcine reproductive and respiratory syndrome virus by blocking viral attachment. Infect Genet Evol 67:78–87
70. López-Gálvez F, Randazzo W, Vásquez A, Sánchez G, Decol LT, Aznar R, Gil M, Allende A (2018) Irrigating lettuce with wastewater effluent: Does disinfection with chlorine dioxide inactivate viruses? J Environ Qual 47:1139–1145
71. Sharma VK, Graham NJ (2010) Oxidation of amino acids, peptides and proteins by ozone: a review. Ozone Sci Eng 32:81–90
72. Schmidt A, Wolff MH, Weber O (2005) Coronaviruses with special emphasis on first insights concerning SARS. Springer Science & Business Media
73. Mizzen L, Hilton A, Cheley S, Anderson R (1985) Attenuation of murine coronavirus infection by ammonium chloride. Virology 142:378–388
74. Alam MS, Takahashi S, Ito M, Komura M, Ono M, Daio C, Sangsriratanakul N, Shoham D, Alam J, Takehara K (2018) Virucidal efficacy of a quaternary ammonium compound with food additive-grade calcium hydroxide towards avian influenza virus and newcastle disease virus on abiotic carriers. Avian Dis 62:355–363
75. McDonnell G, Russell AD (1999) Antiseptics and disinfectants: activity, action, and resistance. Clin Microbiol Rev 12(1):147
76. Knotzer S, Kindermann J, Modrof J, Kreil TR (2015) Measuring the effectiveness of gaseous virus disinfectants. Biologicals 43(6):519–523

77. Yamaguchi Y, Shimodo T, Chikamori N, Usuki S, Kanai Y, Endo T, Katsumata K, Terashima C, Ikekita M, Fujishima A, Suzuki T, Sakai H, Nakata K (2016) Sporicidal performance induced by photocatalytic production of organic peroxide under visible light irradiation. Sci Rep 6:33715
78. Goyal SM, Chander Y, Yezli S, Otter JA (2014) Evaluating the virucidal efficacy of hydrogen peroxide vapour. J Hosp Infect 86(4):255–259
79. Rutala W, Weber D (2008) Healthcare infection control practices advisory committee 2008 guideline for disinfection and sterilization in healthcare facilities, 2008, updated. Available at: https://www.cdc.gov/infectioncontrol/pdf/guidelines/disinfection-guidelines-H.pdf
80. Kariwa H, Fujii N, Takashima I (2006) Inactivation of SARS coronavirus by means of povidone-iodine, physical conditions and chemical reagents. Dermatology 212(Suppl. 1): 119–123
81. Rabenau HF, Kampf G, Cinatl J, Doerr HW (2005) efficacy of various disinfectants against SARS coronavirus. J Hosp Infect 61(2):107–111
82. Weinmann T, Forster F, Von Mutius E, Vogelberg C, Genuneit J, Windstetter D, Nowak D, Radon K, Gerlich J (2019) Association between occupational exposure to disinfectants and asthma in young adults working in cleaning or health services: results from a cross-sectional analysis in Germany. J Occup Environ Med 61:754–759
83. Choi H-Y, Lee Y-H, Lim C-H, Kim Y-S, Lee I-S, Jo J-M, Lee H-Y, Cha H-G, Woo HJ, Seo D-S (2020) Assessment of respiratory and systemic toxicity of Benzalkonium chloride following a 14-day inhalation study in rats. Part Fibre Toxicol 17:5
84. Chang A, Schnall AH, Law R, Bronstein AC, Marraffa JM, Spiller HA, Hays HL, Funk AR, Mercurio-Zappala M, Calello DP (2020) Cleaning and disinfectant chemical exposures and temporal associations with COVID-19Covid-19—national poison data system, United States, 1 Jan 2020–31 Mar 2020. Morb Mortal Wkly Rep 69:496
85. Bracco D, Dubois M-J, Bouali R (2005) Intoxication by bleach ingestion. Can J Anesth 52:118–119
86. Medina-Ramon M, Zock J, Kogevinas M, Sunyer J, Torralba Y, Borrell A, Burgos F, Anto J (2005) Asthma, chronic bronchitis, and exposure to irritant agents in occupational domestic cleaning: a nested case-control study. Occup Environ Med 62:598–606
87. Sawalha AF (2007) Storage and utilization patterns of cleaning products in the home: toxicity implications. Accid Anal Prev 39:1186–1191

Chapter 8
Study on the ANN Forecasting of Epidemical Diseases

Nihar Kanta Sahoo

1 Introduction

The widespread of a disease in a community at a particular period is called an epidemic. It becomes necessary to take effective preventions. This precision of prevention originates from the statistical solutions especially used for forecasting problems. Forecasting the outbreak of epidemics is the leading topic of the research. It delivers information about awareness before taking actions on the influence of an epidemic. The forecasting models use past information from a different angle of studies such as demographic, immunological or geographical data of outbreaks [1]. Usually, epidemic forecast models estimate the growth, peak time, and duration of the epidemics. There are several types of ANN models adopted for forecasting [2]. These models necessitate past epidemiological data set to achieve either short- or long-term forecast. Every model purposes of achieving a generalization mode in forecasting. However, there are significant differences found in high-precision forecast models [3] based on the using of right tools and methodologies. Selection of right tool as well as methods is a challenging task for analysing of epidemic growth. Some models used nonlinearity to find the presence of epidemical dynamics with an exact forecast [4]. Therefore, having the insight to study the forecasting models will be helpful of selecting epidemic forecast method. This chapter delivers a summary on the function of stand-alone ANN and hybrid ANN [5, 6] on epidemical forecasting model. It explains the effect of modelling, performance, accuracy, and limitation of models based on infectious disease outbreaks, which would be fruitful for the analysts.

In year of 2020, the most epidemical disease is COVID-19. Currently, more than 200 countries have been affected by COVID-19. Developing countries like India suffer extremely from the problem of an infectious disease due to the combined effects of existing ecological, social, financial, and demographic factors.

N. K. Sahoo (✉)
Center for Electromagnetics, CSIR-NAL, Bangalore, India

M. Mohapatra et al. (eds.), *COVID-19 Pandemic*, Materials Horizons: From Nature to Nanomaterials, https://doi.org/10.1007/978-981-16-4372-9_8

To implement these measures, data from various sectors need to be analysed, for example, local/government hospital records, climatic, demographic, and environmental factors, social media content, Web search queries, etc., for getting the current medical scenario along with the past data about the disease and the disease information like its symptoms, its spread (duration and carriers), etc., for forming the knowledge base of the diseases. There are different types of network structures. Based on that, MLPFFNN [7] is one of the best-suited methods. This chapter proposes an optimized network architecture using stand-alone MLPFFNN (9–20-1) model to predict the new arrival cases of COVID-19 in the month of July 2020.

2 Basics of ANN

An ANN [7] is a massive parallel-distributed structure formed by a set of neurons. It has a natural ability to forecast obtaining knowledge of past information. It can be used to achieve a task several times faster than the advanced system. The network has some parameters such as weights, bias, transfer functions, learning algorithms, and neurons. The architecture of network depends on the number of layers forming by number of neurons. All neurons are interconnected through weight values and bias inputs. Then, the training algorithm is used to train the network by changing weight values in an orderly manner based on transfer functions to attain the objective. Proper training of the network leads to generalized mode, which provides reasonable outputs beyond the training. Although a neural network cannot produce the solution independently, preferably, it needs to be combined with an engineering approach. In the epidemic forecast, the neural network is capable to work individually if the data are available in social source. ANN offers useful properties such as nonlinearity, input–output mapping, evidential response, contextual information, fault tolerance, VLSI implementation, and neurobiological analogy [8]. It can be easily adjustable to problems and data characteristics. Especially, neural networks are implemented for optimization process, cost-effectiveness, nonlinear mapping for large data sets, etc.

3 Overview of Epidemiology Using ANN

Epidemiology is a branch of medicine, which deals with factors of disease and its possible control [9]. It includes quantitative and analytical techniques, principles based on logical inquiry and procedures for disease management. It determines the allocation and managing of healthcare resources. It also evaluates intervention strategies and the effect of medical services. Mathematical modelling for epidemiology is provided in [10], which helps to develop a model in epidemic situations. The information related to epidemics is crucial for precaution and control, which necessitates developing a model. Forecasting model should be selected based on faster training, accuracy, and efficiency. Among them, ANN is a best-suited method, adaptability to higher-degree nonlinearity, and faster using less computational burden.

This section describes epidemical classifications and ANN models. In [11], a survey explained about diagnostic approaches in medicine based on the application of ANN. It includes image analysis, drug design, biochemical analysis, etc. Dybowski and Gant [12] investigated clinical experiments of diseases using ANN modelling. In [13], deterministic model is developed based on disease control using ANN. Susceptible–infected–recovered (SIR) [14] model evaluates the epidemical transmission rate using ANN. However, neural network is implemented to categorize and define the harshness of diseases in a population [15]. Raja Lakshmi and Mala [16] proposed a radial basis function-based neural network (RBFNN) to diagnose diseases.

Epidemical classification is based on spreading manner that deals with several groups. A group indicates a known pattern, each of which has further refined characteristics to specify the infectious disease correctly. ANN has significant realizations in this epidemic classifications [15]. It also becomes a significant tool for data mining of medical records that can be used for classification and prediction purposes [17]. ANN was implemented for classifying diseases such as dengue fever [18], heart diseases [19], West Nile virus diseases [20], tuberculosis [21], gestational diabetes mellitus [22], swine flu [23], and pancreatic cancer [24]. The forecasting of epidemic models includes the use of ANN, time series analysis, hybrid algorithm data mining [2], and so on. However, ANN epidemic models are extensively accepted for exploration on the risk factors and outbreak size of diseases [25]. The recurrent neural network (RNN) models are usually implemented as a forecasting model against the non-recurrent models. These works based on ANN were helpful for diagnosis and control of epidemics.

4 Complications in ANN-Based Epidemic Model

The development of ANN epidemical model focuses on forecasting using suitable methods. In this forecasting, modelling of ANN depends on data pre-processing, network architecture, inputs, hidden layers, training algorithms, transfer functions, epochs, and performance factors. There should be an optimum balance between all these parameters to get accurate performance.

4.1 Data Pre-processing

In practical, the data are usually incomplete, imbalanced, high-dimensional, and limited. Therefore, data pre-processing is one of the primary processes to pre-process the data for finding the converging performance of the network. It contains transformation, scaling, and normalization. Scaling removes the outliers, transformation transforms into a proper scale, whereas the normalization scales the data in a uniform range (0, 1) or (−1, 1). Binary and linear transformations are used in epidemical classification. The normalization techniques such as z-score, minimax, and sigmoid or soft normalization [7] are applied in this processing. The minimax method is implemented in dengue growth [27]. Sometimes, epidemics have severe impacts within a short duration; continuous data accumulation becomes harmed by under- or over-reporting. Short epidemics data set become insufficient for training and testing. Therefore, random noise can be included to produce new data set. Pasini [26] proposed an equivalent ANN model for the epidemical forecasting with a smaller data set.

4.2 Network Architecture

The architecture of the network contains input nodes, hidden layers, and output nodes, which is the primary factor to determine the network performance. The architecture can be defined based on the mutual information between input and output variables [7]. Too many input nodes or fewer input nodes can directly affect the performance of the network. Therefore, the number of inputs depends on transmission and controlling parameters of disease. Input parameters can be the effect of climate, demographic factors, growth rate, intervention, risk factors, symptoms, and control measures. These data sets are used as input in the forecasting model.

The number of nodes in the hidden layers is likely to simplify the nonlinearity in the epidemic model. The output node of the model predicts incidence, recovery, death rates, and new arrival cases. These outputs depend on the data set needed to exercise the network. Sometimes, infective cases can be the target data of the network, which needs infection incidence data, while death or recovered cases will require mortality or control data.

4.3 Activation Function

The transfer function is also called an activation function. The nonlinearity of the problem with multiple factors and complex relationships used nonlinear activation functions. Formulation of training algorithm changes according to the activation function. The performance of the neural network [8, 28] depends on the function, which provides a degree of nonlinearity. These activation functions are used to perform epidemical forecasting, optimization, classification, pattern recognition, image compression, and so on [29]. There is no thumb rule for the selection of these functions [8]. Therefore, Sibi [30] provided a parametric study on a specific activation function for a specific forecasting model. Sometimes, it has been that more than one functions are used in the same or different layers, which becomes an approach to provide faster training. According to [29], the nonlinear nonnegative functions should be used for the prediction of growth parameters of the diseases, whereas the most commonly used function is the sigmoid (logistic) function for epidemic forecasting model. This function is bounded and differentiable.

4.4 Training Algorithms

Apart from the activation functions and network architecture, the training algorithm is another factor, which can directly affect the performance of the neural network. Few popular algorithms are such as backpropagation, Levenberg–Marquardt, quick propagation, conjugate gradient, competitive learning, and quasi-Newton [7]. The rate of convergence, robustness, and local optima are performance factors of these training algorithms. Backpropagation and LM algorithm [32] are the most popularly used training algorithms. Backpropagation is a gradient descent technique, which has a slow convergence rate but efficient [8, 33] for epidemic forecasting model. On the other hand, the LM algorithm is a comparatively less efficient but faster rate of convergence.

The training process also depends on the number of hidden neurons, learning rate, momentum factor, epochs, and size of data set. These factors can directly affect [31] the training. Correct specification of training parameter is convergence, training time, and generalization. Therefore, hybrid training algorithms are more efficient for improving the performance of the network. The genetic algorithm implementation optimizes the weight values for the faster learning of the neural network which increases the performance of ANN in forecasting [34]. Thereafter, training algorithm minimizes the overall squared error between actual and desired values.

4.5 Under-fitting and Overfitting

Sometimes, under- or overfitting problem arises which can affect the generalize mode of the network. An under-trained model because of insufficient data set produces a higher sum of squared error (SSE). Similarly, overtrained happens when the network fits for training and produces poor result beyond the training. Therefore, the researcher's suggestion is to alternate the algorithm and architecture or pre-process the data set. Some researchers used the following mathematical expression [35] to estimate the under-fitting.

$$\varepsilon_1 = \frac{SSE_k - SSE_{k-1}}{SSE_k} \leq \varepsilon_1^* \tag{1}$$

The calculation of MSE is for both training (MSE_T) and validation (MSE_V) data set and then uses the following equation to avoid the overfitting [36]

$$\varepsilon_2 = \frac{MSE_T - MSE_V}{MSE_T} \leq \varepsilon_2^* \tag{2}$$

The precision of ε_1 and ε_2 is problem-dependent. The cross-validation technique is also implemented for solving overfitting. Several techniques are there for cross-validation such as leave-one-out, leave-p-out, k-fold, hold-out, and Monte Carlo. K-fold converts randomly the data set into k-partitions. The kth subset is used as a test set, and the model is trained using other partitions. Normally, tenfold cross-validation is used.

4.6 Hybrid ANN Epidemic Forecast Model

Epidemic model based on ANN helps to observe the spreading disease [37]. Zhang et al. [8] provided a model based on heuristics and simulations. However, ANN requires a larger database for its proper training. The intension of hybridization is for the advantage over traditional methods and heuristics. The hybrid concept deals with a combination of two different algorithms to achieve better performance. Infectious and non-infectious illnesses have been determined to adopt hybrid ANN in obtaining good accuracy. Basheer et al. [31] recommended that ANN can be hybridized. For the pandemic forecast, the other models or statistical methods can be integrated with ANN. Algorithm hybrid executes the learning method further effective across standard algorithms, and data hybrid is imperative for the heterogeneous data structure. Technology hybrid with ANN produces more reliable platform and makes more accelerated pandemic forecasting and analysis. It solves puzzles of the machine in fact of both software and hardware. Cloud-based technology [38] realizes the ANN model to investigate medical data for assessing and grading epidemics. Therefore, the hybridization of ANN is justified.

Moreover, hybrid ANN model carries other nonlinear forecasting models like fuzzy logic, ARIMA, and logistics regression. Generally, these methods are coupled with ANN for high-precision forecasting. The hybrid method overwhelms the deficiency of stand-alone methods by reducing overall error and converging time. Hybrid ANN model challenges other algorithms such as weight fixing algorithms, training algorithms, error minimization techniques, and time-dependent functions. The application of evolutionary algorithms [39], genetic algorithms (GA) [40], evolutionary programming, particle swarm optimization [35], ant colony optimization, bird mating optimizer (BMO) [41], and bat algorithm [42] enhances the ANN training in the epidemic forecasting model.

Arifianto et al. [43] developed a model by combining the group method data handling (GMDH) with the neural network to forecast malaria outbreaks in South East Asia. Belciuf and Gorunescu [44] have attended a similar approach. They realized GA weight training for an MLPNN to forecast the detection and recurrence of breast cancer. Gan et al. [45] used the combination of grey model (GM) and backpropagation algorithm to determine the germination of hepatitis B. The performance of this combination has an advantage over the all-conventional approach of GM.

The combinational performance of autoregressive integrated moving average (ARIMA) method and nonlinear autoregressive recurrent neural network (NARNN) is highly acceptable. This combined method performs better than individual models in forecasting schistosomiasis. Yan et al. [46] proposed a combination of seasonal ARIMA and with generalized regression neural network to predict bacillary dysentery. The similar hybrid algorithm is also used for the prediction of tuberculosis. The limitations of stand-alone forecast methods are almost overwhelmed by hybridization. An analogous approach can be enhanced by hybridizing more techniques such as data, algorithm, and technology in an epidemic forecasting model. This model can reach accuracy.

4.7 Overall Comparison of ANN on Epidemical Model

ANNs have substantial advantages over conventional statistical approaches. The advantages are based on the type of problem and data, training time, requirement of resources, parameterization, and adaptivity. In [47, 48], a few points have been declared on the performance of the neural network. The deterministic nature of the data series, sampling variability, and hybridization of methods tends to be quite accurate and outperforms the individual methods. A comparison of ANN alternatives with SARIMA forecast technique is provided [49]. It is proved that RBFNN, ERNN, and BPNN exceed SARIMA in terms of short memory series. Further, the performance of ANN outperforms the nonlinear regression models in forecasting dengue outbreak [27]. On the pandemic study of malaria [50] and infectious diarrhoea in China [51], the ANN outperforms the support vector regression (SVR), random forest regression (RFR), and multivariate linear regression (MLR) methods.

4.8 Coronavirus Disease 2019 (COVID-19)

A novel virus was found at the end of 2019 in China. World Health Organization (WHO) officially announced this virus as COVID-19. COVID-19 is a double-stranded RNA (ribonucleic Acid) virus that depends on other organisms. This virus is transmitted through droplet infections or FECO/oral route. It can enter the body of the human through the nasal cavity, eye, and mouth. The virus goes into the respiratory tract by the mucus membrane. This virus receives the nutrients from the normal cells of the body that weakens the immune system. It affects the respiratory organs, alters the normal process of lungs, and shows symptoms such as fever, dry cough, sore throat, shortness of breath, lethargy, respiratory malfunction, severe headache, head riling, malaise, and loss of test and smell. It also affects other vital organs like brain, heart, kidney, and lever by the help of bloodstream. Aetiology deals with the cause of the disease. The disease spreads by an affected person to others. Aetiology includes travel history. Initially, it stays under the people who came only from affected countries. Nowadays due to higher spreading rate, it includes inter-country, interstate, inter-district, as well as inter-village communications. Secondly, aetiology deals with those persons who are contacted with suspected cases.

Growth rate depends on the risk factors. Risk factors deal with low immune system categories such as child, pregnant women, old age people, low immune system human, health personal, police, fourth-grade workers and people living in red zone area. Thereafter, its diagnostic and evaluation are under consideration. History collections and physical examinations (head to toe) come under the diagnostic process, and evaluation starts with high-grade fever, increases respiratory rate, and alters BP and heart rate. Then, clinical diagnostic comes for the testing process of the virus. Clinical diagnostic prefers the swab test, especially the nasal swab test.

There are three steps of medical treatment: (i) COVID care centre, (ii) designated COVID care centre, and (iii) designated COVID hospital and three stages for COVID patients such as mild (asymptomatic or little symptom), moderate (patients required oxygen during their treatment stage), and severe (required ICU). The three-step treatment deals with each state of patients. In a survey, it has been known that 84% are in mild condition, 11% are moderate, and only 5% are severed in condition.

4.9 Detection of COVID-19 Using ANN

The first patient from China was hospitalized on 12 December 2019. There has been around more than 150 countries affected by this virus by the end of June. Initially, the proper control parameters and precautions have been unknown which causes severe spreading over the world.

There is an insufficient amount of COVID-19 test kits provided to the hospitals. It is essential to develop an automatic detection system as a quick alternative diagnosis option. Z. Pamuk et al. [52] suggested the use of three convolutional neural network-based models such as ResNet50, InceptionV3, and Inception-ResNetV2. These models can recognize the coronavirus pneumonia-infected patient using chest X-ray radiographs. The performance of pre-trained ResNet50 is about the 98% accuracy based on classification, whereas InceptionV3 and Inception-ResNetV2 are having 97% and 87%, respectively. A similar approach has been proposed by the Alexander Wong et al. [53] using convolutional deep neural network. Jun Xia et al. [54] suggested COVID-19 detection neural network (COVNET). This model extracts visual features from volumetric chest CT examinations for the detection of COVID-19.

5 Proposed Model for COVID-19 Case Prediction

This chapter works on a neural network model to forecast the arrival of the new case of COVID-19 in the forthcoming days [55]. The proposed model is a multi-layer perceptron (MLP) neural network with error backpropagation algorithm. It contains one hidden layer and an output layer. The sigmoid transfer function and linear transfer function are used in the hidden layer and output layer, respectively. The training of the network uses the parameters mentioned in Table 1. The input parameters are a number of days, average low temperature, average humidity, hygiene index, stringency index, percentage of migrant workers displaced, number of test per thousand, percentage of the middle-age population (age between 20 and 45), and percentage of old age population (age after 65). The target of the network is new case arrival per day from 1 March 2020 to 25 July.

This COVID-19 spreading becomes more powerful in its proper weather condition. Therefore, average low temperature and humidity are the climatic factors taken as the input of the network. Hygiene index is taken as an input parameter, which depends on the per capita income, cleanliness, sanitization facilities, and awareness. The percentage of age categories is an important factor in growth rate due to low or high immune system. Nation-wise lockdown became a major precaution to weaken the spreading rate of COVID-19, which depends on the stringency index. This index indicates that India had toughest lockdown measures in the world at a 100 score since 22 March. It observes containment policies such as school and workplace closings, public events and transport, and stay at home policies. A higher index value means a higher level of stringency. The growth rate of COVID-19 in few states becomes higher due to a larger number of migrant workers displaced. As a conservative number, at least 500 million migrant workers displaced by road, rail, and airways from their places since March onwards. The percentage of migrant worker displaced is taken as an input for network training.

6 MLPFFNN

Figure 1 shows the network architecture of the proposed model. Here, f is a mapping function (*tanh)* used by the proposed model that maps the inputs $I_1(n), \ldots, I_k(n)$ to the new arrival cases $Y(n)$ in each day n and k is the number of inputs. The model output is

$$Y(n) = u_o(n) \tag{3}$$

$$u_o(n) = \sum_{j=1}^{h} \left(w_j z_j(n)\right) + b \tag{4}$$

Table 1 Pandemic of COVID-19 (As on 25 July): first case detected (FCD), avg. temp. (AT), humidity (H), lockdown start (LDS), death percentage (DP), per capita income (PCI) in $, hygiene index (HI), number of test/100 (NOT), total number of test (TT), population (P)

Country	FCD	AT	H	LDS	DP	PCI	HI	NOT	TT	P
USA	19-Jan	15	53	7-Apr	3.49	59,928	73.02	36.96	52,522,208	330,758,784
Spain	31-Jan	14	72	14-Mar	8.9	39,800	92.75	41.05	6,320,836	46,752,556
Russia	31-Jan	−5.52	85	30-Mar	1.6	26,470	69.7	51.93	26,610,623	145,926,781
UK	27-Jan	6	81.25	23-Mar	15.33	45,350	84.25	29.41	14,291,673	67,841,324
Italy	30-Jan	10.5	75	21-Feb	14.29	42,290	91.59	33.71	6,468,375	60,472,650
Brazil	25-Feb	22	80	8-Apr	3.6	15,850	70.1	0.62	4,911,063	212,368,566
France	24-Jan	8	78.1	9-Mar	16.7	41,464	86.94	12.73	2,982,302	65,255,646
Germany	27-Jan	12	71.6	9-Mar	4.5	54,560	83.06	37.57	7,418,812	83,750,665
Turkey	21-Jan	16	52	17-Mar	2.4	27,640	62.81	20.11	4,489,360	84,222,640
Iran	19-Feb	18	40.2	28-Mar	5.3	21,050	69	8.53	2,302,634	83,853,830
India	30-Jan	26	67.00	24-Mar	2.33	7680	58.9	1.3	15,849,068	1,378,270,651
Peru	6-Mar	14.5	85	15-Mar	4.7	13,710	63.3	3.29	2,183,763	32,912,133
China	17-11-19	12.1	56.5	23-Jan	N	18,170	62.52	N	N	1,439,323,776
Canada	13-Feb	−5.24	70	15-Mar	7.84	47,590	85.7	36.38	3,717,483	37,700,059
Belgium	4-Feb	10	83.4	17-Mar	6.67	51,740	80.46	50.55	1,514,046	11,583,327
Saudi Arabia	2-Mar	30	46.3	23-Mar	1.02	55,840	73.5	17.75	2,946,928	34,742,883
Mexico	28-Feb	24	59.3	1-Apr	11.2	19,340	62.09	1.21	896,124	128,759,156
Netherlands	27-Feb	10	83	5-Apr	11.67	56,890	85.86	17.89	851,885	17,130,183
Chile	3-Mar	15.2	71	16-Apr	2.6	21,190	73.21	21.43	1,485,711	19,095,344
Pakistan	26-Feb	21	70	21-Mar	2.1	5860	56.8	1.88	1,844,926	220,321,573
Ecuador	29-Feb	17.8	78	16-Mar	6.9	11,420	61.8	3.05	221,152	17,608,034
Belarus	1-Apr	7	79.7	N	0.7	19,240	70.9	41.03	1,241,624	9,449,669
Sweden	31-Jan	6	77.8	N	7.2	54,030	90.24	20.78	751,213	10,092,027

(continued)

Table 1 (continued)

Country	FCD	AT	H	LDS	DP	PCI	HI	NOT	TT	P
Switzerland	5-Mar	9	78.6	19-Mar	5.7	68,820	90.93	41.06	758,836	8,647,311
Portugal	2-Mar	17.5	85	4-Mar	3.4	32,680	83.1	66.1	1,528,600	10,199,983
Singapore	23-Jan	26.8	80	3-Apr	0.0005	94,670	89.29	32.69	1,170,049	5,845,014
Bangladesh	7-Mar	25.9	65.8	31-Mar	1.3	4570	53.2	1.18	1,101,480	164,497,521
UAE	29-Jan	26.8	61.3	6-Apr	0.5	75,440	67.14	0.8	4,776,904	9,876,291
Poland	11-Jan	19	78.3	24-Mar	3.9	30,010	87.2	17.83	2,068,983	37,851,214

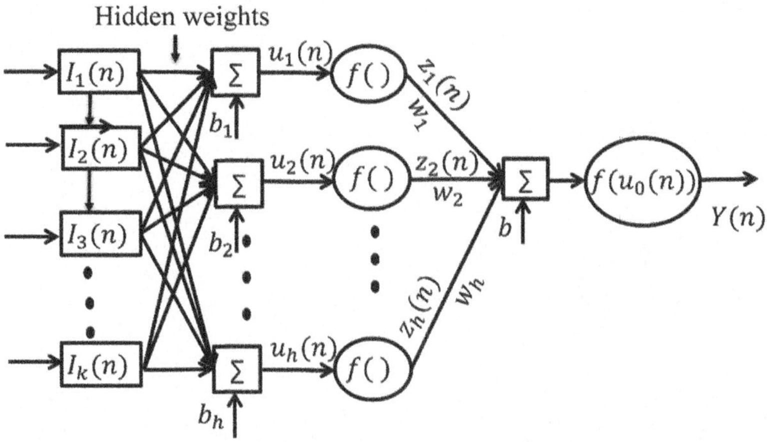

Fig. 1 Proposed MLPFFNN model for new arrival case prediction

$$z_j(n) = f(u_j(n)) \tag{5}$$

$$u_j(n) = \sum_{i=0}^{k} w_{ij} I_k(n) + b_j \tag{6}$$

In the above equations, $u_j(n)$ is the input to the *jth* hidden neuron, $z_j(n)$ is the output of the *jth* hidden neuron, $u_o(n)$ is the output of the network, w_{ij} is the weight from the *ith* input to *jth* hidden neuron, w_j is the weight from *jth* hidden neuron to the output, b_j is the hidden bias, *b* is the output bias, and *h* is the number of hidden neurons. *f* is a sigmoid transfer function at each hidden neuron.

The performance of the model is measured by mean square error (MSE):

$$MSE = \frac{1}{M} \sum_{n=1}^{M} \left(\hat{Y}(n) - Y(n)\right)^2 \tag{7}$$

where $\hat{Y}(n)$ and $Y(n)$ are the desired and network output values, respectively, for the *nth* sample and *M* is the number of data samples. The network performance is adjusted through backpropagation learning rule. The weight is adjusted using the following formulations.

$$\begin{aligned} w &\leftarrow w + \Delta w \\ \Delta w_{ij}(n) &= \eta \delta_j(n) Y(n) \end{aligned} \tag{8}$$

For a neuron *j* located at the output layer, the local gradient is

$$\delta_j(n) = \frac{b}{a}\left[\hat{Y}(n) - u_o(n)\right][a - u_o(n)][a + u_o(n)] \tag{9}$$

For a neuron j at the hidden layer, then the local gradient is

$$\delta_j(n) = \frac{b}{a}\left[a - z_j(n)\right]\left[a + z_j(n)\right]\sum_k \delta_j(n) w_j(n) \tag{10}$$

7 Result Discussion

The proposed network contains 9 inputs, 20 hidden neurons, and 1 target. A parametric study has been done on the performance based on number of data and hidden neurons. A close approximation has been found using the network architecture 9–20-1. The proposed model uses cases of the first 104 days for training and testing. Then, the trained network forecasts new arrival cases of the next 43 days. The training covers 70%, whereas testing covers 30%. Figure 2 shows the training plot of the 9–20-1 proposed network for prediction of the new cases of COVID-19. MSE drops below 10^{-2} within 500 epochs.

Figure 3 shows a comparison of new arrival cases from 13 June 2020 to 25 July 2020. There is a significant deviation of 10,000 to 5000 cases between the predicted curve and the original curve from 13 June to 3 July, whereas the matching becomes closer after 3 July up to 25 July of less than 3000 cases which indicates that the performance network is under the tolerable limit. The input data have been collected from so many anonymous sources, which might be the cause of deviation between predicted and original curves.

The similar network is used by taking the input values from 1 March 2020 to 30 June 2020 (122 days). The data of 122 days are used to train the same network which is used then to forecast new arrival cases of the next 25 days. Figure 4 shows a close approximation of the maximum deviation of 1500 from 5 July to 20 July

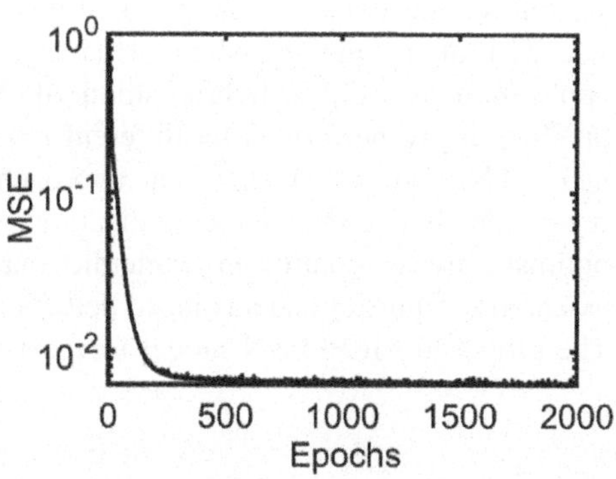

Fig. 2 Training curve of proposed MLPFFNN model

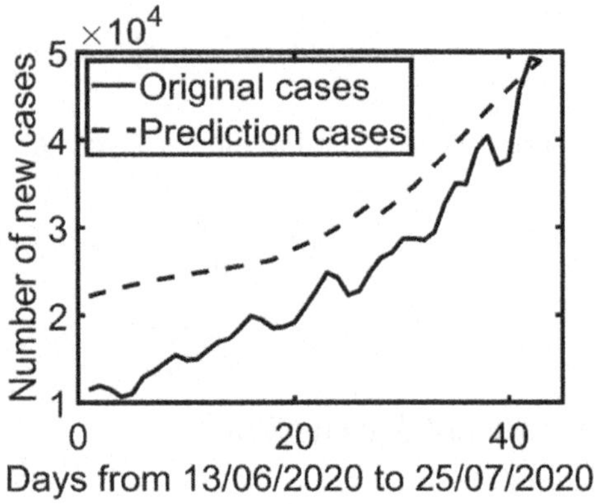

Fig. 3 Comparison of MLPFFNN model prediction and original cases

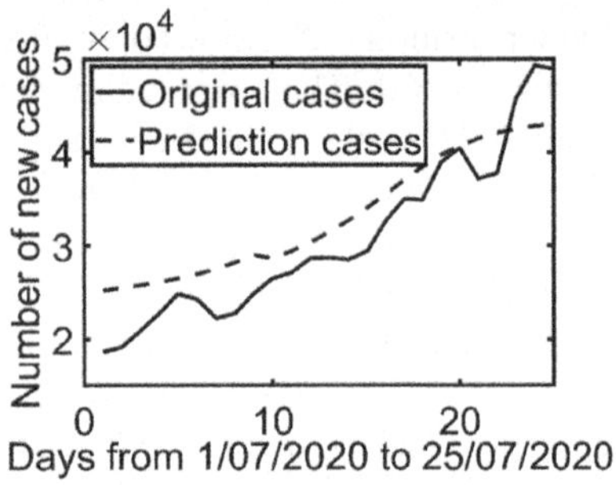

Fig. 4 Comparison of MLPFFNN model prediction and original cases

2020 (15 days), whereas a deviation of fewer than 5000 cases is seen first and last five days. Due to the more training data, the approximation is closer than Fig. 3.

8 Conclusion

The forecasting is essential in deciding intervention and control strategies. Therefore, the detailed survey on different model characteristics will assist the selection of a suitable model. This chapter presented a brief summary of the application as well as hybridization of ANN in the epidemic forecast. Several predictions are performed by different models on the nature of pandemic diseases using ANN and other statistical approaches. The use of ANN is not limited to prediction, but it includes classification, optimization, parameter estimation, and optimal disease control in epidemic management. The use of ANN is being essential for quicker and advanced detection that can reduce the chance of infection. The proposed MLPFFNN model forecasts new cases with some deviation limit.

References

1. Wu JT, Cowling BJ (2018) Real-time forecasting of infectious disease epidemics. Hong Kong Med J Xianggang Yi Xue Za Zhi 24(Suppl 6, 5):26–29
2. Bharambe AA, Kalbande DR (2016) Techniques and approaches for disease outbreak prediction: a survey. In Proceedings of the ACM symposium on women in research 2016, Indore, India, Mar. 2016, pp 100–102 https://doi.org/10.1145/2909067.2909085
3. Tabataba FS et al (2017) A framework for evaluating epidemic forecasts. BMC Infect Dis 17 (1):345. https://doi.org/10.1186/s12879-017-2365-1
4. Satish S (2017) Epidemic disease detection and forecasting: a survey. 3
5. Razi MA, Athappilly K (2005) A comparative predictive analysis of neural networks (NNs), nonlinear regression and classification and regression tree (CART) models. Expert Syst Appl 29(1):65–74. https://doi.org/10.1016/j.eswa.2005.01.006
6. Paliwal M, Kumar UA (2009) Neural networks and statistical techniques: A review of applications. Expert Syst Appl 36(1):2–17. https://doi.org/10.1016/j.eswa.2007.10.005
7. Haykin SO (2008) Neural Networks and Learning Machines, 3rd edn. Pearson, New York
8. Zhang G, Patuwo BE, Hu MY (1998) Forecasting with artificial neural networks: the state of the art. Int J Forecast 14(1):35–62. https://doi.org/10.1016/S0169-2070(97)00044-7.
9. Ahrens W, Pigeot I (eds) (2014) Handbook of Epidemiology, 2nd edn. Springer-Verlag, New York
10. Canzani E, Lechner U (2015) Insights from modeling epidemics of infectious diseases—a literature review. 8
11. Amato F, López A, Peña-Méndez EM, Vaňhara P, Hampl A, Havel J (2013) Artificial neural networks in medical diagnosis. J Appl Biomed 11(2):47–58. https://doi.org/10.2478/v10136-012-0031-x
12. Kareem SS, Pathak Y (2016) Chapter 20—Clinical Applications of Artificial Neural Networks in Pharmacokinetic Modeling. In: Puri M, Pathak Y, Sutariya VK, Tipparaju S, Moreno W (eds) Artificial Neural Network for Drug Design, Delivery and Disposition. Academic Press, Boston, pp 393–405
13. Rao VSH, Kumar MN (2010) Estimation of the parameters of an infectious disease model using neural networks. Nonlinear Anal Real World Appl 11(3):1810–1818. https://doi.org/10.1016/j.nonrwa.2009.04.006
14. Correia AM, Mena FC, Soares AJ (2011) An Application of the SIR model to the evolution of epidemics in portugal. In: Dynamics, games and science II, Berlin, Heidelberg, pp 247–250. https://doi.org/10.1007/978-3-642-14788-3_19
15. Waidyarathne KP, Samarasinghe S (2014) Artificial neural networks to identify naturally existing disease severity status. Neural Comput Appl 25(5):1031–1041. https://doi.org/10.1007/s00521-014-1572-6
16. Rajalakshmi V, An GS, Mala H (2016) Software aided diagnosing of diseases using RBF based neural networks [RADD]. Biomed Res 27(3). Accessed: 06 Aug 2020. [Online]. Available: https://www.alliedacademies.org/abstract/software-aided-diagnosing-of-diseases-using-rbf-based-neural-networks-radd-4558.html
17. Shouman M, Turner T, Stocker R (2012) Using data mining techniques in heart disease diagnosis and treatment. In: 2012 Japan-Egypt conference on electronics, communications and computers, Mar 2012, pp. 173–177. https://doi.org/10.1109/JEC-ECC.2012.6186978
18. Laureano-Rosario AE et al (2018) Application of artificial neural networks for dengue fever outbreak predictions in the northwest coast of Yucatan, Mexico and San Juan, Puerto Rico. Trop Med Infect Dis. 3(1). https://doi.org/10.3390/tropicalmed3010005
19. Khemphila A, Boonjing V (2011) Heart disease classification using neural network and feature selection. In 2011 21st International conference on systems engineering, pp 406–409. https://doi.org/10.1109/ICSEng.2011.80

20. Ghosh D, Guha R (2010) Use of genetic algorithm and neural network approaches for risk factor selection: A case study of West Nile virus dynamics in an urban environment. Comput Environ Urban Syst 34(3):189–203. https://doi.org/10.1016/j.compenvurbsys.2010.02.007
21. Elveren E, Yumuşak N (2011) Tuberculosis Disease Diagnosis Using Artificial Neural Network Trained with Genetic Algorithm. J Med Syst 35(3):329–332. https://doi.org/10.1007/s10916-009-9369-3
22. Muller PS, Sundaram SM, Nirmala M, Nagarajan E (2015) Application of computational technique in design of classifier for early detection of gestational diabetes mellitus. Appl Math Sci 9:3327–3336. https://doi.org/10.12988/ams.2015.54319
23. Tarle B, Jena S(2017) An artificial neural network based pattern classification algorithm for diagnosis of heart disease. In 2017 International conference on computing, communication, control and automation (ICCUBEA), Aug 2017, pp 1–4. https://doi.org/10.1109/ICCUBEA.2017.8463729
24. Bartosch-Härlid A, Andersson B, Aho U, Nilsson J, Andersson R (2008) Artificial neural networks in pancreatic disease. Br J Surg 95(7):817–826. https://doi.org/10.1002/bjs.6239
25. Wahyunggoro O, Permanasari AE, Chamsudin S, Utilization of neural network for disease forecasting. 6
26. Pasini A (2015) Artificial neural networks for small dataset analysis. J Thorac Dis 7(5):953–960. https://doi.org/10.3978/j.issn.2072-1439.2015.04.61
27. Husin NA, Mustapha N, Sulaiman MN, Yaakob R (2012) A hybrid model using genetic algorithm and neural network for predicting dengue outbreak. In: 2012 4th Conference on data mining and optimization (DMO), Sep. 2012, pp 23–27. https://doi.org/10.1109/DMO.2012.6329793
28. Karlik B, Olgac AV (2011) Performance analysis of various activation functions in generalized MLP architectures of neural networks
29. Isa IS, Saad Z, Omar S, Osman MK, Ahmad KA, M, Sakim HA (2010) Suitable MLP network activation functions for breast cancer and thyroid disease detection. In: Modelling and simulation 2010 second international conference on computational intelligence, Sep 2010, pp 39–44 https://doi.org/10.1109/CIMSiM.2010.93
30. Sibi P, Jones SA, Siddarth P (2005) Analysis of different activation functions using back propagation neural networks. 47(5)
31. Basheer IA, Hajmeer M (2000) Artificial neural networks: fundamentals, computing, design, and application. J Microbiol Methods 43(1):3–31. https://doi.org/10.1016/S0167-7012(00)00201-3
32. Shirangi MG, Emerick AA (2016) An improved TSVD-based Levenberg–Marquardt algorithm for history matching and comparison with Gauss–Newton. J Pet Sci Eng 143:258–271. https://doi.org/10.1016/j.petrol.2016.02.026
33. Reynaldi A, Lukas S, Margaretha H (2012) Backpropagation and Levenberg-Marquardt Algorithm for Training Finite Element Neural Network," in *2012 Sixth UKSim/AMSS European Symposium on Computer Modeling and Simulation*, Nov. 2012, pp. 89–94 https://doi.org/10.1109/EMS.2012.56.
34. Karegowda AG, Manjunath AS, Jayaram MA (2011) Application of genetic algorithm optimized neural network connection weights for medical diagnosis of PIMA Indians diabetes. https://doi.org/10.5121/IJSC.2011.2202
35. Yaghini M, Khoshraftar MM, Fallahi M (2013) A hybrid algorithm for artificial neural network training. Eng Appl Artif Intell 26(1):293–301. https://doi.org/10.1016/j.engappai.2012.01.023
36. Ghiassi M, Saidane H (2005) A dynamic architecture for artificial neural networks. Neurocomputing 63:397–413. https://doi.org/10.1016/j.neucom.2004.03.014
37. Soemsap T, Wongthanavasu S, Satimai W (2014) Forecasting number of dengue patients using cellular automata model. In: 2014 International electrical engineering congress (iEECON), Mar 2014, pp 1–4 https://doi.org/10.1109/iEECON.2014.6925876.
38. Maithili A, Kumari DRV, Rajamanickam MS (2012) Neural networks cum cloud computing approach in diagnosis of cancer. 2(2):8

39. Yao X (1999) Evolving artificial neural networks. Proc IEEE 87(9):1423–1447. https://doi.org/10.1109/5.784219
40. Jia W, Zhao D, Shen T, Su C, Hu C, Zhao Y (2020) A new optimized GA-RBF neural network algorithm. Comput Intelli Neuroscience 13. https://www.hindawi.com/journals/cin/2014/982045/. Accessed 06 Aug 2020
41. Askarzadeh A, Rezazadeh A (2013) Artificial neural network training using a new efficient optimization algorithm. Appl Soft Comput 13(2):1206–1213. https://doi.org/10.1016/j.asoc.2012.10.023
42. Khan K, Sahai A (2012) A Comparison of BA, GA, PSO, BP and LM for Training Feed forward Neural Networks in e-Learning Context. Int. J. Intell. Syst. Appl. 4(7):23–29. https://doi.org/10.5815/ijisa.2012.07.03
43. Arifianto A (2014) Malaria incidence forecasting from incidence record and weather pattern using polynomial neural network. Int J Future Comput Commun 60–65. https://doi.org/10.7763/IJFCC.2014.V3.268
44. Belciug S, Gorunescu F (2013) A hybrid neural network/genetic algorithm applied to breast cancer detection and recurrence. Expert Syst 30(3):243–254. https://doi.org/10.1111/j.1468-0394.2012.00635.x
45. Gan R, Chen X, Yan Y, Huang D (2015) Application of a hybrid method combining grey model and back propagation artificial neural networks to forecast hepatitis B in China. Comput Math Methods Med 26.. https://www.hindawi.com/journals/cmmm/2015/328273/. Accessed 06 Aug 2020
46. Yan W, Xu Y, Yang X, Zhou Y (2010) A hybrid model for short-term bacillary dysentery prediction in Yichang City, China. Jpn J Infect Dis 63(4):264–270
47. Makridakis S, Hibon M (2000) The M3-Competition: results, conclusions and implications. Int J Forecast 16(4):451–476. https://doi.org/10.1016/S0169-2070(00)00057-1
48. Crone SF, Hibon M, Nikolopoulos K (2011) Advances in forecasting with neural networks? Empirical evidence from the NN3 competition on time series prediction. Int J Forecast 27 (3):635–660. https://doi.org/10.1016/j.ijforecast.2011.04.001
49. Zhang X, Liu Y, Yang M, Zhang T, Young AA, Li X (2013) Comparative study of four time series methods in forecasting typhoid fever incidence in China. PloS One 8(5):e63116.https://doi.org/10.1371/journal.pone.0063116
50. Rismala R, Liong TH, Ardiyanti A (2013) Prediction of malaria incidence in Banggai Regency using evolving neural network. In 2013 InternationalcConference on technology, informatics, management, engineering and environment, Jun. 2013, pp 89–94.https://doi.org/10.1109/TIME-E.2013.6611970
51. Wang Y, Li J, Gu J, Zhou Z, Wang Z (2015) Artificial neural networks for infectious diarrhea prediction using meteorological factors in Shanghai (China). Appl Soft Comput 35:280–290. https://doi.org/10.1016/j.asoc.2015.05.047
52. Narin A, Kaya C, Pamuk Z (2020) Automatic detection of coronavirus disease (COVID-19) using X-ray Images and deep convolutional neural networks. *ArXiv200310849 Cs Eess*, Jul. 2020, Accessed 06 Aug 2020. [Online]. Available: http://arxiv.org/abs/2003.10849
53. Wang L, Wong A (2020) COVID-Net: a tailored deep convolutional neural network design for detection of COVID-19 cases from chest X-Ray Images. ArXiv E-Prints 2003. arXiv:2003.09871
54. Li L et al (2020) Artificial Intelligence distinguishes COVID-19 from community acquired pneumonia on Chest CT. Radiology 200905. https://doi.org/10.1148/radiol.2020200905.
55. Car Z, Baressi Šegota S, Anđelić N, Lorencin I, Mrzljak M (2000) Modeling the spread of COVID-19 infection Using a multilayer perceptron. Comput Math Methods Medi. https://www.hindawi.com/journals/cmmm/2020/5714714/ (accessed Aug. 06, 2020).

Chapter 9
Simulation Studies Related to COVID-19 Pandemic

E. V. Bhavya and Balamati Choudhury

1 Introduction

As per the latest report from WHO, more than 78 million people are infected and 1.7 million people lost their lives due to COVID-19 as on December 2020. The latest findings across the world proves that this pandemic disease spreads through the close contact of COVID-19 positive persons or by touching the contaminated objects or surfaces. The COVID-19 contamination happens mainly through the virus filled saliva or through respiratory secretions.

While there are a lot of research and works are happening today around the world to invent medicine for curing this disease, the current ways to avoid contracting COVID-19 are to keep social distancing, use effective masks or cloths to cover mouth and nose and maintain personal hygiene by frequently washing hands. When social distancing is difficult to implement in public places, office, etc., wearing masks as per required standard is an important measure to get protected and to protect others.

While scientists and doctors are still in the mode of discovering new features of this virus, the recent study shows, this disease is air born as well since it transmits through aerosols. Aerosols are small droplets released while coughing or sneezing and it has an ability to suspend in the air for extended periods of time. These aerosol particles can be a potential course for COVID, if this particle reaches human body during inhalation. As a result, it is critical that all health personnel doing these

E. V. Bhavya (✉) · B. Choudhury
Center for Electromagnetics (CEM), CSIR-National Aerospace Laboratories (NAL), Bangalore 560017, India
e-mail: balamati@nal.res.in

and

Academy of Scientific and Industrial Research (AcSIR), Ghaziabad, Uttar Pradesh 201002, India

M. Mohapatra et al. (eds.), *COVID-19 Pandemic*, Materials Horizons: From Nature to Nanomaterials, https://doi.org/10.1007/978-981-16-4372-9_9

medical operations use specialized airborne safety measures, such as wearing suitable personal protective equipment (PPE) and face masks.

COVID-19 is largely transmitted through virus loaded droplets and aerosols that are produced inside the respiratory gland of an infected individual will be exorcized from the mouth and nose during normal coughing as well as sneezing and also while talking loudly. The fate of these droplets is determined by the rival effects of inertia, gravity and evaporation. Droplets which are larger than the critical size contaminate surrounding surfaces by settling faster than they evaporate. Droplets minor than this critical size dissolve faster than they settle, hence already formed droplet nuclei can stay in the air for hours and may become the primary cause for the transmission over long distances.

From air–mucous interaction through liquid sheet fragmentation, turbulent jets, droplet evaporation and deposition, to flow-induced particle dispersion and sedimentation, each droplet experiences a multitude of complicated events. The relevance of the transmission process, as well as the strategies, devices, and practices used to prevent respiratory infections, are all based on fluid dynamics principles. These include necessary precautions such as hand washing, personal hygiene and wearing face masks, to fogging machines, proper ventilation and even practices such as social distancing.

There are multiple outbreaks reported for COVID-19 in public spaces, including restaurants [1], hospitals, nightclubs, holly spaces or office spaces where people may get into close contacts. Recent study indicates that aerosol transmission cannot be ruled out as cause of these outbreaks, mainly in overpopulated and poorly ventilated indoor spaces where COVID contracted people come in contact with non-infected people. While additional studies are carrying out to inspect such occurrences and evaluate the significance of COVID-19 spread, we recommend simulation studies to understand the COVID-19 transmission behaviours in different scenarios such as through air, risk of transmission with and without various type masks, effectiveness of social distancing, design of negative pressure room and ventilator design etc. A detailed literature review on some of the simulation studies related to this field is given below.

2 Simulation of Ventilation System of Hospital Room

With no proven treatment/medicine and daily increase in percentage of healthcare professional infected via transmission by novel coronavirus is putting an massive stress on healthcare infrastructures around the world. As a result, there is an immediate need for low-cost testing and isolation rooms in high-population-density areas to prepare for a worst-case community spread scenario. To isolate the infected person from others and to take the samples, negative pressure rooms and booths are used in hospitals. A specially ventilated room is used as negative pressure room, where the operating pressure is kept lower than in the surrounding area so that there is no considerable escape of contaminated air. By using computational fluid dynamics (CFD) study one can understand the contamination dispersion characteristics and also can be used to design a modular negative pressure room that is also easy to manufacture. CFD analysis optimizes the airflow pattern and temperature distribution to accomplish a better thermal control level. Engineers devised and assessed many ventilation design concepts for this study in order to determine the most effective for eliminating contaminated air from the isolation room and the best choice for physical prototype. In this pandemic situation using CFD analysis helps to better understand the COVID-19 dispersion characteristics as well as helps in building easy to manufacture cost-effective ventilation systems for hospital rooms.

During past years, numerous studies have concentrated on computational models utilizing fluid dynamics to explore flow analysis and the associated transmission of contamination in hospital space for various ventilation frameworks [1–5]. The major consideration in these studies were the assessment of the impacts of ventilation and negative pressure rooms in spreading the infection. The HVAC design will always aid to control negative pressure inside isolation rooms and to safeguard hospital staff, patients and companions. The isolation room maintains negative pressure to decrease the flee of aerosols, and the high air exchange rate can quickly remove aerosols, thereby eliminating the spread of infectious aerosols to the outdoors.

After SARS outbreak Li et al. [6] did a review on the effect of ventilation in the construction environment on the spread of infectious agents in the air. They did a vast study on the major literature databases between the time span of 1960 and 2005, and then based on the title, abstract and a set of other criteria finally selected 40 original studies. They established a review team consisting of medical and engineering specialist in the fields of microbiology, medicine, epidemiology, indoor air quality and building ventilation. Out of 40 the panel systematically assessed 10 selected studies with regard to the association between building ventilation and the transmission of airborne infection. They found that there is sufficient and adequate evidence to prove the relationship between building ventilation and air circulation and the spread of infectious diseases such as measles, tuberculosis, chickenpox, influenza, smallpox and SARS.

Kermani [7] analysed the airflow pattern and aerosol transmission in a single-bed hospital room. Aerosol spread from the patient's respiratory organs and the total thermal comfort of the isolation room are discussed in his paper. The proposed model includes a bed, a patient, a doctor, a wardrobe, a lamp, medical equipment and an inlet and exhaust system. He considered forced and natural ventilation, and the flow of bacterial trace produced by infected patients. The proposed room geometry is shown in Fig. 1. According to the ASHRAE 170 standard, the ventilation rate of healthcare facilities is 6 ACH (air changes per hour). The air comes through the ceiling diffuser (entrance) in room at a temperature of 20 °C and then exits through a grill (exit) installed on the ceiling as shown in Fig. 1. The extension area of the entrance and exit is small to rule out numerical uncertainty. A lamp is considered as the heat source in the proposed model and is placed amongst the entrance and exit, and the medical equipment was placed in the corner of the room.

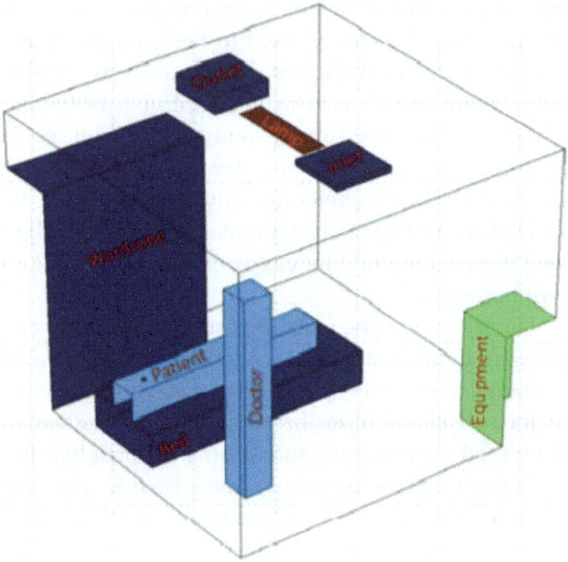

Fig. 1 Hospital room layout (reused from Alireza Kermani 2015)

Moreover, a consistent heat flux will be there in the room produced by the doctor and infected person.

He utilized turbulent flow and heat transfer calculations in COMSOL Multiphysics software to get airflow owing to natural and induced convection in the hospital room. These physics solve the air-coupled Navier–Stokes and continuity equations and the thermal convection and diffusion equations. The turbulence is solved by using the stable and stable k-ω (k-ω) turbulence model. Figure 2 shows the temperature distribution and velocity vector near the doctor and patient. After computing the temperature and velocity distribution particle tracing module in simulation software is used to analyse the spreading of bacteria in the room due to coughing. He used massless particle design for this study with a total of 250 bacterial particles. Through this research, he tried to estimate the fraction of bacteria escaping the room through the ventilation system.

In his study, he concluded that less than 30 s after coughing, no bacteria left the room where 8% of the bacteria remained in the room after 300 s, which in turn can cause infection spread. Figure 3 shows the movement of bacteria at 30, 60, 180 and 230 s after coughing. Thirty seconds after coughing, most bacteria leave the room through exhaust. Still, about 10% of them stayed in the room and shifted to the bottom corner of the room in the next 30 s. Figure 3c indicates that, in the next 180 s, they are gradually travelling parallel to the floor and towards the patient again. Approximately 2% of the remaining bacteria exit room 220 s after coughing. The remaining 8% of the bacteria as shown in Fig. 3d may contaminate the whole room and surge the risk of airborne contaminations.

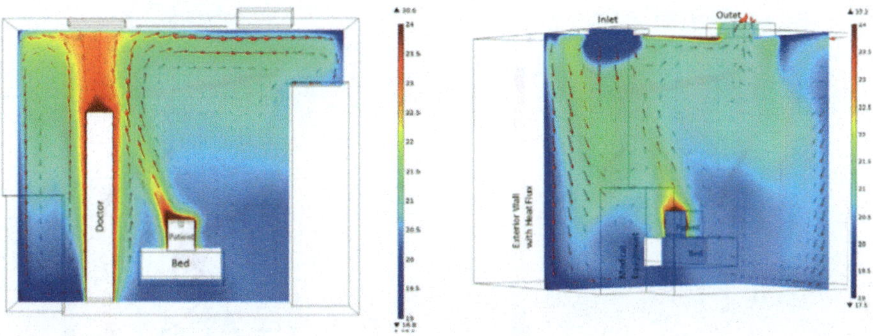

Fig. 2 Temperature distribution and velocity vector in the room. The colour legend corresponds to the temperature (°C) (reused from Alireza Kermani 2015)

In another study Mahajan et al. [8] studied about the airflow simulation of an isolation room using CFD technique. A three-dimensional model of an isolation room of size 4 × 4 × 2.5 m^3 comprises of stationary man and patient is modelled in SolidWorks software. The isolation room is discretized hexahedrally using finite volume approach with blocking methodology and is simulated using ANSYS FLUENT tool. The flow physics of airflow is simulated around the stationary man and the patient using steady-state simulation and the velocity, pressure and temperature behaviour were observed by plotting contours.

Balocco [9] did a hospital ventilation simulation to investigate possible contaminant exposure. He started with the hypothesis that patients could have a risk for airborne disease in isolation rooms due to either poorly planned or wrongly functioning ventilation system. The paper investigates the conditions that particles discharged from patients during coughing can have an increased possibility of interfering with the patient's breathing and vice versa though Multiphysics approaches along with critic review of literature results and experimental evidences. Since there are various practical difficulties such as long lead time for legal approvals, hospital technicians' low cooperation, unable to do spot test to collect the real experimental measurements, etc., leads to the importance of using CFD-FEM simulation to validate the experimental evidences. In this study as model was defined relating droplet dispersion due to cough and sneeze that can carry virus and carried out CFD-FEM transient simulation based on Multiphysics approach.

In this article, Group considered 10 μm particle and are contagious up to 2-m distances. As per the report from [10, 11], particle with above-mentioned dimension stay in the air up to 491 s while moving with a trajectory of 1.5 m. Particles with dimension greater than 50 μm cannot remain in air for a longer period of time hence the chance of infection through inhalation is rare. Besides, particles of the size of 1.0 μm evaporate very quickly. In this proposed model team used Cunningham Slip Correction (Cc) to predict the drag force between a fluid and a particle moving through this fluid [12–14] because the fluid is no longer continuous when particle diameters become small [12, 13, 15]. In this scenario, the drag coefficient on each

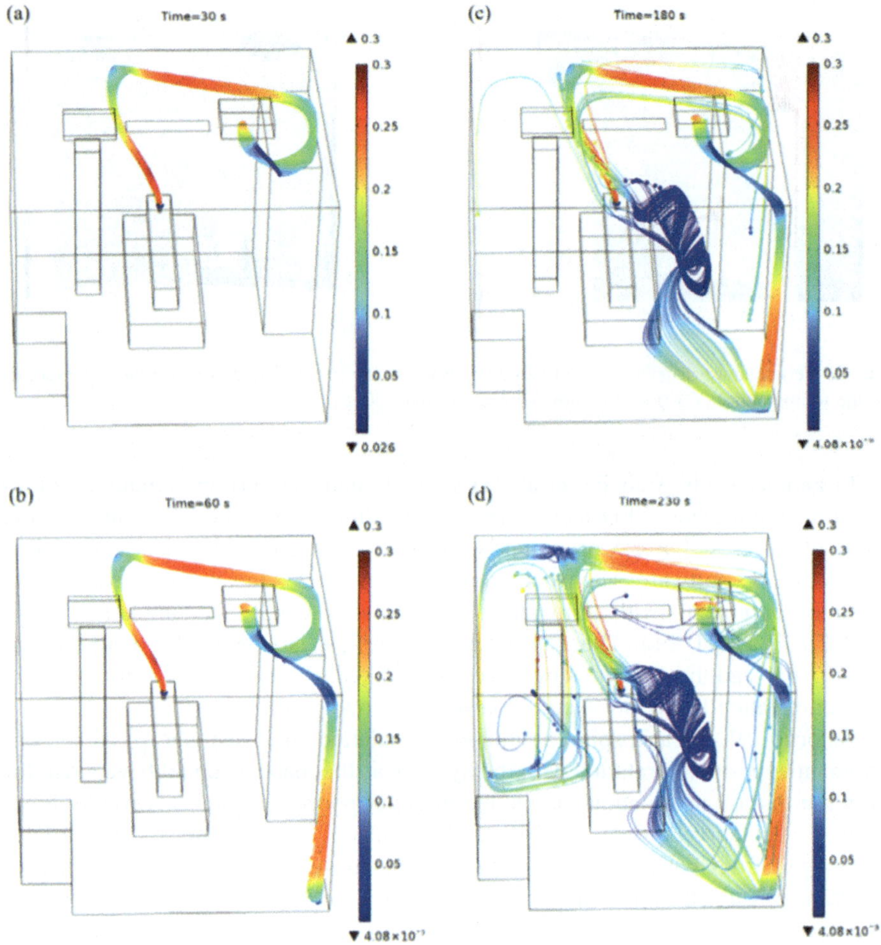

Fig. 3 Particle tracing showing the motion of bacteria particles at 30, 60, 180 and 230 s after patient coughing. Particle colour corresponds to velocity (m/s) (reused from Alireza Kermani 2015)

particle must be divided by the Cunningham correction factor and the correction factor is greater than 1, which means drag coefficient goes down for these effective particles.

Using CAD database, 3D model of the isolation room was designed. Team used SolidWorks 2009 commercial design software and solid-modelled the inlet high induction air diffuser by progressively varying its shape considering tilt and directionality of its fins. CFD-FEM simulations were carried out by using COMSOL Multiphysics software (Fig. 4).

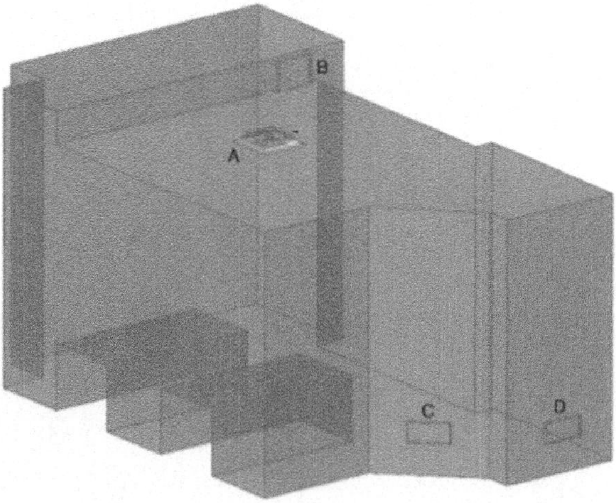

Fig. 4 The 3D geometry of the isolation room with the air inlet (A) and air return (B, C, D) diffusers (reused from Balocco2011)

Simulation was conducted for two patients' coughing and breathing processes that lasts for 60 s to study airflow patterns and effectiveness of ventilation system inside the room. From the simulation it has been observed that the particle density is more in the breathing area (near source) at about 10 cm, and the velocity field mainly rise to the ceiling due to the combined effect of the ventilation with the temperature gradient (Fig. 5). The particle tracing results highlights the fact that the position of the air return diffusers and central high induction air supply are not successful in eliminating particles and viruses at the patient's breathing area. Due to coughing, the diffusion flux and concentration of particles highlight the position of particles with a diameter of about 510-μm during the cough as shown in Fig. 5. These trajectories in Fig. 5 state the initial momentary position of these particles overlapping with the oral cavity surface of the coughing patient.

This study provides useful indications for infection control and effective design and optimization of ventilation systems in the studied isolation room. This study also helps to predict the best way to select type and position of the high inlet air diffuser in order to reduce the mixing between supply air and the air in the room. A mean velocity of 0.25 m/s is obtained at the patients' bed which comes under the recommended threshold value and can be used to predict the contagious zone in the room. The result also predicts the exact location of air diffuser to be close to the floor and among and behind the head of two patients. The residual bio-aerosol concentration was also studied for the open-door condition and the result for both open- and closed-door condition suggest the best safety distance between the beds to control the transmission of infection in patients as well as in medical staff and visitors.

This study mainly focusses on use of ventilation system in the isolation room especially in the zone between two beds to improve efficiency of contamination removal, though the current ventilation system is not adequate to control the contamination due to coughing and sneezing. Result highlights the deficiency of

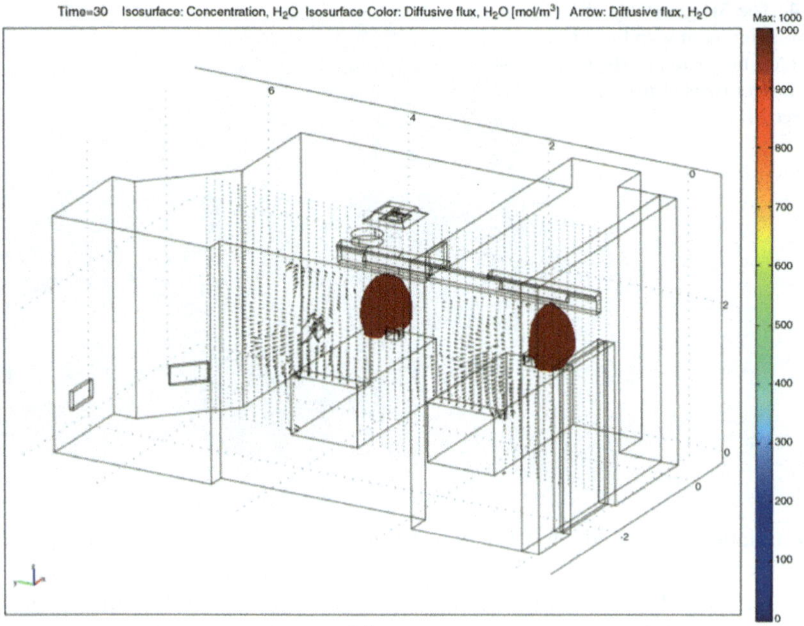

(a)

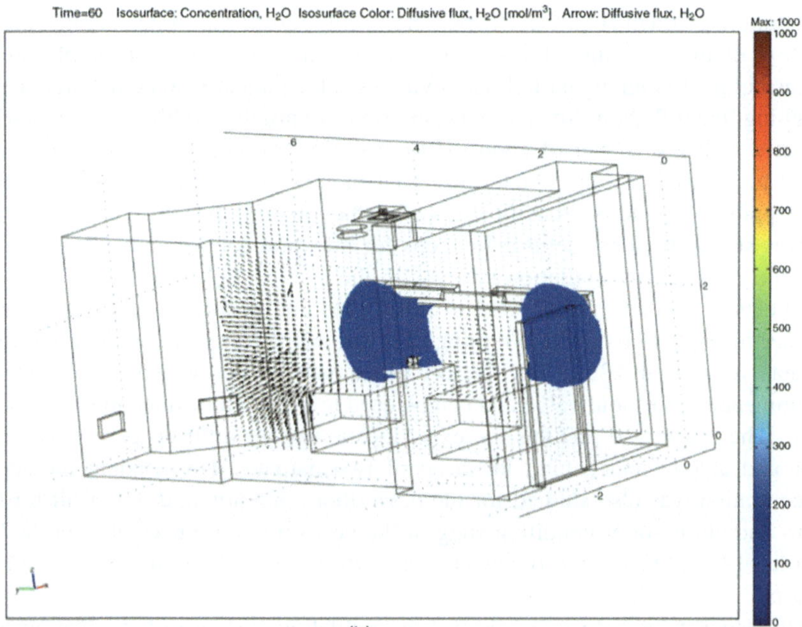

(b)

Fig. 5 Particle concentration and diffusive flux, model_3, at X **a** 30 s and **b** 60 s of transient simulation (reused from Balocco 2011)

current ventilation system's capability to control contamination through open door. This paper also highlights this usage of cost-effective CFD-FEM simulation to determine ventilation system's efficiency by replicating real scenarios and extending its application to evaluate efficiency in real scenarios as well. This method also has multiple application in other private and public places.

Jacob et al. [16] in his research paper tried to optimize the ventilation plan towards contaminant suppression in the isolation room. A CFD-FVM analysis is done for an isolation room by using Navier–Stokes and energy equation with the help of appropriate boundary conditions. During CFD simulation, patient body is replaced with a semi-cylindrical shape with constant heat source. Using CFD solver, team simulated the bed position and air inlet position in the isolation room for an infectious and immune-suppressed patient.

These two configurations were simulated to study the velocity and temperature profiles of the isolation room. The study suggests the best position to place the immune-suppressed patient and SARS infected patient to reduce the transmission of the contamination, results suggest to place the infected patient near the exhaust to flush out the droplet through the exhaust as soon as they generated and immune-suppressed patient near the air supply to avoid getting infection through the air.

"Safe ventilation rate" has been determined by Jiang et al. [17] to eliminate hospital-based airborne virus infections and prevent cross-infection of severe acute respiratory syndrome (SARS). They used a simulation method to reproduce three actual cases, among them when SARS patients were hospitalized in a nearby room, a group of hospital occupants reportedly infected or not. This work offers a method for exploring the effective ventilation rate from an engineering perspective.

Computational fluid dynamics (CFD) and multi-zone model-based simulations were carried out to understand the dilution level of SARS virus filled aerosols during these three cases along with a series of measurements. A safe ventilation rates (dilution level) for SARS infection and non-infection were determined based on these scenarios and that for a SARS patient to eliminate the air bone viral infection is to dilute the air emitted from the patient by 10,000 times with clean air.

According to the investigation, they concluded that keeping the SARS virus constant above a certain level will lead to a higher probability of infection. The study concluded that when the dilution relative to air is less than 1000 times and the average exhaust volume is 0.3 m^3/h per person, the risk of pollution is high, while the dilution is higher than 10,000 times, resulting in a low risk of infection. At the same time, since infection is a very complex process and involves many factors, more research in this area is needed to establish a clear boundary between safe dilution rate and dangerous dilution rate. Therefore, these results indicate that the use of simulation tools to reproduce actual infected and non-infected cases is an effective technique for determining safe ventilation rates to maintain a non-infected building environment. In addition, it provides a way to study the necessary ventilation rate from an engineering perspective.

3 Simulation Related to Social Distancing and Respirator Mask

In order to get proof and gain visibility into the "social distancing" Feng et al. [18] used a computational fluid-particle dynamics (CFPD) model for simulating the instantaneous migration, condensation/evaporation and deposition of SARS-CoV-2 filled droplets released by coughing under diverse environmental wind speeds and relative humidity (RHs). The initial droplet diameter ranges from 2 to 2000 μm, and the wind speed ranges from 0 to 16 km/h, representing different wind forces from stable air to moderate breeze, and considering the relative humidity of 40% and 99.5%. Feng et al. also investigated the effect of mask on minimizing spread of droplets released during coughing. A closed rectangular parallelepiped space was reconstructed, in which there were two human samples set up virtually and placed at distance of 1.83 m and 3.05 m, respectively. Well-known Euler–Lagrange-based multiphase flow model is applied to study the behaviours of virus filled droplets produced by coughing. Key behaviours studied are droplet's movement, variation in size and deposition. The methodology they used in this work is listed below [18].

Methodology

1. 3D modelling and Meshing—a closed rectangular parallelepiped space was reconstructed, in which there were two human samples set up virtually and placed at distance of 1.83 m and 3.05 m, respectively.
2. Numerical modelling—Euler–Lagrange-based multiphase flow model is applied to study the behaviours of virus filled droplets produced by coughing. Key behaviours studied are droplet's movement, variation in size and deposition.
3. Boundary and initial condition

   - Transient cough-jet airflow waveform—modelled the waveform using the experimental data drawn from study conducted on 25 subject's cough patterns
   - Initial size distribution of cough droplet—the initial droplet diameter ranges from 2 to 2000 μm
   - Boundary conditions—when a droplet is deposited on the boundary or escapes from the computational domain, the size and spatial position of the droplet are recorded.
   - Initial condition

     - Wind speed—0 to 16 km/h
     - Air inlet temperature—27 °C
     - Humidity—RH = 40%, for ideal condition, and RH = 99.5% for upper limit.

4. Numerical calculation

   To model the transient airborne propagation of cough droplets transported by ambient airflow under condensation and/or evaporation, ANSYS Fluent 2019 is utilized. The highest droplet time step is 1.0e−5 s, while the flow time step is 1.0e−3 s [18].

The ambient wind enhances the secondary flow through the recirculation in the computational domain. Micro-droplets deposit on both human bodies and head regions by following the airflow streamlines well even with the 3.05-m (10-feet) separation distance and some of them travels a distance more than 3.05 m due to wind triggering potential risk to nearby people. Relative humidity has an effect on droplet dispersion as RH increases it will in turn increases the droplet size which will result in deposition of these droplets on both humans and ground. This study shows that the six-feet social distancing standard may not be sufficient to limit interpersonal aerosol transmission, because suspended droplets are affected by convective effects and can be removed from a person's cough/sneeze in less than 5 s. The sneeze can also be transferred to another person, under complicated environmental wind and relative humidity conditions. Also, it reports the behaviour of virus filled droplet released during coughing and it includes the location and particle size at different instances from t = 1.0 s to t = 15.0 s. When the ambient wind velocity is zero, droplets can only receive momentum and energy from the cough jet. Large droplets can be found to travel faster and remain more concentrated than small droplets. On the contrary, as the ratio of surface area to volume increases, the small droplet loses its initial momentum and kinetic energy more quickly due to the viscous dissipation effect of resistance.

Therefore, they disperse very quickly in static air. This study proves that under the existing social distancing policy of 1.83 m (6 feet), droplets can still be transmitted to the head area of the human model standing 6 feet from the transmitter. Thus, even for ideal static air conditions, existing social distancing policies may not be 100% safe. When wind velocity, Vin = 5.5 m/s, wind convection dominates the small droplet trajectory. Specifically, the droplets are confined in an area whose width is roughly equal to the width of the shoulder. Meanwhile, the horizontal recirculation flows to the centre line between two people who are separated by six-feet distance. In addition, the main convection transfers additional momentum and kinetic energy to the droplets and accelerates the droplets to move quickly along the airflow streamline to the head of a healthy person standing 6 feet away from the person who is coughing. Compared with static air, it has a recirculation effect in the vertical direction, and some droplets move backwards and stay around the person who is coughing. Hence, the ambient wind will make the transport dynamics of aerosols further complicated and may offer them with higher kinetic energy and make them spread farther in the air.

To explore the efficiency of mask, a N95 mask model was recreated and kept adjacent to the virtual human model who coughs. To study the worst-case situation of inappropriate mask usage the average gap between the profile and the edge of the N95 mask was deliberately magnified by 1.8 cm. For the simulation with the N95 mask, the riskiest case of Lsd = 1.83 m (6 feet), Vin = 5.5 m/s and RH = 99.5% was picked. The droplet transport dynamics are visualized at various time stations for comparisons without N95 mask. While there are still cough droplets that the mask cannot catch, the total number of cough droplets dispersed in the air is much lower compared to the case without a face mask. With a mask, the droplets in the air are moderately low. The initial time they enter the free air stream is somewhat delayed. The mainstream airflow can still follow these tiny droplets and enter the virtual individual on the right. Therefore, it can be concluded that wearing a mask can essentially decrease the spread of cough droplets in the air even if it is not properly sealed with the face. It is suggested that people wear face coverings to minimize the gap between faces to maximize the effect. In order to slow down the spread of the COVID-19 virus through the air, even though a "social distance" policy of roughly 1.83 m (6 feet) is suggested, it still needs to be carefully studied. By using the CFPD method to visualize the trajectory and fate of SARS-CoV-2 filled droplets under numerous environmental circumstances and to simulate the condensation/evaporation effect between surrounding water vapour and droplets, this study found that 1.83 m (6 feet). The social distancing policy is the "minimum requirement", and due to the complexity of the environmental wind conditions, it is not enough to avoid exposure to SARS-CoV-2. These assumptions do not take into account the sneezing droplet cloud, which may span approximately 8 m (27 feet). Therefore, the height of safe social distance depends on different factors, so it is strongly suggested that people wear masks and other face shields in public places. The main inferences from the study are as follows: (1) coughing COVID-19 carriers can release micron-sized virus droplets, which can still survive in the air, keeping healthy people away from the source (6 feet) and far away (10 feet) in a static air environment. (2) The influence of wind on the transport and deposition of droplets is complicated and heavily reliant on the wake pattern and local secondary flow strength between two virtual humans and the stability of the wind. To be sure, the current six-foot social distancing policy is not enough to protect people from SARS-CoV-2 exposure caused by coughing and surrounding wind. (3) A higher RH = 99.5% results in a higher fraction of deposition on the human body and the ground, which is not inherently correlated with a higher risk of exposure. A higher RH = 99.5% can enhance the condensation effect, and the size of the cough droplet will continue to grow during the propagation in the air until the partial pressure of the droplet surface is equal to the saturation pressure of water vapour. Conversely, RH = 40% triggers the evaporation of water in the cough droplet, which results in a decrease in droplet size, which may result in a longer suspension in the air. Though the cough droplet depositions on the human body can be reduced by longer social distances, there are still SARS-CoV-2 laden droplets that can append or deposit on the healthy human near the head area. The suspension of tiny droplets in the air can be greatly decreased even when wearing facial masks in an unrealistically loose state while coughing.

Lei et al. [19] used CFD simulation and infrared imaging technology to evaluate the leakage of the face seal of the respirator. They used CFD simulation methods to predict the leakage between the N95 filter mask respirator (FFR) and the head mould, and used infrared camera (IRC) methods to verify the CFD method. The CFD method is used to calculate the leak position and the "filter-end seal leakage" (FTFL) ratio of 10 head moulds and 6 FFRs. The calculated geometry and leakage gap are determined by analysing the contact simulation results between each headform-N95 FFR combination. The volume grid is constructed using a mesh generation method developed by the author. The breathing air passes through the FFR filter media and the leakage gap. These leakage gaps are zones where no seal is formed around the FFR. The effectiveness of the CFD method was verified by comparing the facial temperature and leakage location measured by IRC with eight subjects. Most leakage occurs in the nose (40%) and right (26%) and left cheek (26%). The findings also suggest that when using N95 FFR (no exhalation valve), the skin temperature in the area near the lips increases and can affect the thermal comfort.

The breathing rate and viscous resistance coefficient of the FFR filter media directly change the FTFL ratio, whereas the flow has no effect on the FTFL ratio. If the limitation can be overcome, the recommended CFD method is a promising alternative to studying FFR leakage. This research developed a method for studying the internal flow in the volume formed between the FFR and the head mould surface (FFR dead space) and the flow outside the FFR based on earlier work [20]. The CFD method is used to simulate the airflow and heat transfer on the face. An algorithm for generating mesh flow field for CFD simulation is developed. Calculated the facial temperature profile over time to determine the location of the leak. The face temperature and leak location in the experiment and simulation were compared for verification.

Ten FE head forms were reconstructed from the digital models of six-N95 FFRs using the method developed by Lei et al. [21]. In every head form geometry, six regions namely forehead, left cheek, right cheek, chin, neck and back of the head were considered. Facial and jugular regions have multilayer structures in which the skin layer is at the head form surface and the bone layer is at the innermost level of the head form [20, 22]. The conditions under which almost all inhaled and inhaled air pass through the filter media define a proper fit. If air leaks through the boundary between the face and the surface of the respirator, a leak will occur. All through exhalation, the breathing air will flow out of the nostrils and enter the dead corner defined by the innermost surface of the respirator, where it partially touches the face. During inhalation, dead space air enters the nostrils, creating a negative pressure field, which makes the air to move from the exterior to the inside of the mask. Therefore, the airflow field comprises three areas: between the head form and the respirator, inside the filter media and outside the respirator. The CFD simulation includes four parts: creating the meshed area of the airflow field, defining the mathematical model of flow and heat transfer, choosing the appropriate solver and analysing the temperature, pressure and velocity fields.

Some of the assumptions they considered during the research were: (i) only nasal breathing; (ii) for heat transfer issues, only conduction and convection are considered because radiation and water evaporation were ignored; (iii) breathing airflow was not hindered by ears or back of the head; (iii) there were no FER variations and no head movement; and (iv) No deformation of the respirator during the CFD simulation. Possible error that causes the difference between simulation and experiment results include the contributions of the above-mentioned assumptions, the difference between the subject's face and head morphological models, numerical errors, and experimental errors. In this study, Lei et al. discovered that majority of leaks occur in the nose and cheek regions. 40% leak appeared near nose and 26% leak appeared near left and right cheek areas. The results also revealed that when using N95 FFR without exhalation valves, there was an increase in skin temperature near the lip, which could be related to thermal discomfort.

In a study, Oestenstad et al. [23] found that leakage from the nose, cheeks and chin responsible for 53%, 14% and 34% of the total leakage, respectively. An ongoing report presented that there is more leakage in the cheeks (40%), less leakage in the nose (37%) and leakage in the chin (23%) [24]. These are not in line with the trend of this research for CFD simulations or infrared images from the human body. In the human body, the nose is usually the obvious leakage part, and the chin is the least common leakage part. This may be because of different subjects, respirators and methods of identifying the leak.

An article by Zhang et al. [25] proposed an improved filter mask respirator (FFR) design to improve the wearer's comfort during low-intensity work. The improved FFR aims to reduce dead zone temperature and CO_2 levels through active ventilation fans. Reverse modelling is used to establish a 3D geometric model of the FFR; then, computational fluid dynamics (CFD) simulation is introduced to study the flow field. According to the simulation results, the improved FFR ventilation fan can adapt to the flow field well when placed in the correct blowing direction. When the fan blows inward, the streamlines are distributed in a cup shape, which perfectly matches the shape of the FFR and the face.

The optimized flow field controls the CO_2 volume percentage in the dead zone of the enhanced FFR. Furthermore, an experimental prototype of the improved FFR was tested to verify the simulation. The wireless temperature sensor detects temperature changes within the prototype FFR. Compared with the ordinary FFR without a fan, the dead zone temperature is reduced by 2 K. The infrared camera (IRC) method is used to clarify the temperature distribution of the outer surface of the prototype FFR and the wearer's face, thereby significantly reducing the surface temperature. The simulated internal and external temperature results are consistent with the experimental results. Therefore, adding an inward blowing fan on the outer surface of the N95 FFR is a feasible method to reduce the CO_2 concentration in the dead zone and improve the temperature comfort.

4 Antiviral Mask Simulation

4.1 Materials Used for Antiviral Property

Face masks have become part of our life in the fight against the coronavirus, to help slow the spread of the deadly outbreak. Though commonly used masks are not effective to stop viral infections, mask technology is relatively advanced to produce mask with effective protection.

The nonwoven material in the mask filters the virus, but the lack of capability to kill the virus makes the mask prone to cross-infection which in turn converts it to a supplementary source of infection once after discarded. Hence an efficient and effective protective mask should ideally have both filtering capability and antiviral effect at the same time.

Medical masks and personal protective equipment are used to efficiently filter the droplets, respiratory secretions and body fluids. The medical protective masks are made considering the end user comfort, so these masks are created using multiple nonwoven layers, including functional wet-resistant nonwoven layer, melt blown nonwoven layer and skin-friendly nonwoven layer. Interception, inertial impact and electrostatic deposition are the three main filtering mechanisms which are primarily used. Filtration and particle characteristics are the parameters mainly used to determine the protection effectiveness of the regular protective masks. Key filtration characteristics includes thickness, packing density, fibre diameter and charge of filed nonwoven layers and particle characteristics include diameter, density and velocity.

Current advancements in nanotechnology open a wide scope in antiviral mask production by successfully evaluating antiviral nanomaterial and incorporating it in to the mask technology to reduce the virus transmission. An antiviral mask can be made by integrating the antiviral nanomaterial in the fibre or nonwoven fabric material in the commonly used mask. Both organic and inorganic materials can be used as the functional element for this purpose [26]. Antiviral personal protective devices including face masks are gaining attention of both industrialists and academicians and various researches are in progress for this area. This section details the recent studies and findings in antiviral agents and relevant results via simulation with the mask. Improving antiviral capability can directly correlate the efficiency of the mask and mitigate the risk of cross-infection or secondary infection while using or managing the mask. Current study also indicates the grater applicability of nanotechnology to transform the design and effectiveness these protection devices.

4.1.1 Silver-Based Antiviral Nanoparticles

Silver, an inorganic material which is known for its anti-pathogen behaviours and also comes up with a great anti-microbial property, can be considered as antiviral agent. When the virus comes in contact with a silver surface, the silver nanoparticle

(Ag NPs) interacts with the outer layer of the virus thereby preventing it to penetrate into the host cell. The antiviral property of Ag NPs is mainly attributed to the average particle size. A lot of studies are already conducted to understand the antiviral property of silver nanoparticle. Orlowski et al. [27] reported the synthesis of Ag NPs with a particle size of 33 nm, successfully manage the herpes simplex virus type 2 (HSV-2) infection in mice by hindering the adhesion of the virus to host cells. Average particle size of the nanoparticle effects the antiviral property along with this to enhance the antiviral action, a few therapeutic agents can also be used as the surface ligands for Ag NPs. Li et al. [28] synthesized Ag with Oseltamivir (Ag@OTV) NPs with a typical size of 3 nm by using OTV as a surface modifier. Ag@OTV solution was used to culture the cells infected with influenza virus (H1N1), and the cell survival rate was 90%, it continued higher than that of bare AG MPs (65%). Adding OTV ligands enhanced the anti-infection capability of Ag NPs. Ag@OTV could successfully hinder H1N1 influenza by generating virus-induced apoptosis of host cells. Likewise, other therapeutic agents (such as amantadine [29], zanamivir [30], and aminoadamantane [31]) were also investigated with Ag NPs to boost the antiviral activity.

Even other silver compounds apart from silver nanoparticles, act as effective antiviral agents. While considering the antiviral capability of silver nanoparticle, yet there is a genuine challenge in combination of silver NPs with fibres, and their integration with personal protection equipment. Surface coating can be used as an effective technology for this application. Tang et al. [32] tried to integrate the silver nanoparticle on silk by using surface coating technology. As a result of Plasmon resonance effect of Ag NP, Ag NP shows an exceptional pathogen destroying capability and is visually recorded by a colour change. When the silk fibre decorated with silver nanoparticles comes into contact with E. coli specimen, more than 99% of E. coli specimen were killed. When coated by Ag NPs, other fibre materials (such as polyester [33], cotton [34] and chitosan [35]) can also significantly stimulate antibacterial activity. However, so far, there are few research results and evidence on the antiviral properties of fibres modified with silver nanoparticles, and this still needs to be focussed in a broader arena.

4.1.2 Gold-Based Nanoparticles (Au NPs)

Au NPs have exceptional biocompatibility, stability and capability to bind to biological ligands (bioconjugation), that are all closely related to the application of antiviral materials. It has been recognized that the mechanism of Au NP inhibiting the virus is based on blocking the combination of virus particles and cells, thereby inhibiting the attachment/entry of the virus and controlling the spread of the virus between cells.

In another study, Li et al. [36] manufactured BNA conjugated networks of gold nanoparticles (DNA-Au NPs) to enhance the specificity of gold-based antiviral materials. This material exhibits excellent antiviral property in opposition to respiratory syncytial virus (RSV). Once the DNA-Au NPs network and RSV virus and cells are cultured together, the cell survival rate exceeds 90%. This DNA-Au NPs network forms a protecting layer on the cell membrane to inhibit virus infection, thus stopping the attachment and entry of the virus, budding and spreading between cells. Diverse forms of gold nanoparticles have dissimilar antiviral characteristics and mechanisms. Bawage et al. [37] proposed the antiviral mechanism of gold nanorods (45 nm × 10 nm) against RSV. In the 2.5 μg/mL content of gold nanorods, the survival rate of RSV-infected cells was 82%. Gold nanorods inhibit viral infections mainly by inducing cellular immune responses.

To diminish the toxicity of Au NPs and enhance their performance, Carja et al. proposed a new method [38]. By accumulating gold nanoparticles (3.5 nm) on large-scale double hydroxide layers (LDHs, 150 nm), micro-nano-hybrid materials (Au NPs/LDHs) were constructed. These hybrid materials show exceptional antiviral ability at dilute state also, and the cell survival rate after hepatitis B virus (HBV) infection exceeds 90%. The gold nanoparticle from the mixture directly interacts with virus and traps the virus in the cells and prevents it from spreading between cells. Nevertheless, they are not commonly used in personal protective equipment because of their high cost.

4.1.3 Copper-Based Nanoparticles

Since copper oxide nanoparticles are a good candidate for antibacterial materials because of their nominal price, great stability and broad antibacterial properties [39, 40], it has also been studied by researchers to evaluate its fitment as an antiviral agent. The study shows copper oxide nanoparticle can use as a potential antiviral agent because its capability to destroy and degrade virus' genome. Borkow et al. [41] stated the creation of antiviral respiratory protective face mask by impregnation of copper oxide nanoparticles (CuO NPs) into an N95 mask so as to investigate the relevance of copper oxide nanoparticle in respiratory mask. The selected N95 mask was composed of four layers in which the inner layer and outer layer were composed of different fibre fineness. The presence of evenly distributed CuO NPs in the masks destroy the virus which were remained in the mask. By coating the copper oxide nanoparticle with N95 mask makes it more efficient and improves the antiviral effect five orders of magnitude.

4.1.4 Carbon-Based Materials

Carbon atoms can take different forms to become various allotropes, such as 0D carbon dots (CDs), 1D carbon nanotubes (CNTs), 2D graphene and 3D diamond. Different studies were conducted to evaluate the anti-microbial effect of carbon allotropes and turn out the unique antibacterial effect comes from their physical and chemical properties.

From these allotropes two-dimensional graphene oxide (GO) has shown excellent anti-pathogen characteristics compared to other allotropes. In one of the studies

Ye et al. [42] investigated the broad-spectrum antiviral activity of GO against pseudorabies virus [PRV, a DNA virus] and porcine epidemic diarrhoea virus [PEDV, an RNA virus]. Go and rGO's' unique single-layer structure and surficial negative charges give rise to their interesting antiviral properties. When GO concentration is adjusting to 6 μg/mL in medium, cell infection caused by PRV and PEDV can be restricted to the magnitude of two orders. The negatively charged GO electrostatically reacts with virus which leads to destruction of sharp edges and single-layer structure of the virus. While there is controversy about GO's antiviral mechanism, Sametband et al. [43] stated that GO prevents herpes simplex virus type1(HSV-1) infections. Furthermore, it is still an unsolved problem to use carbon-based antiviral agent along with fibres without deviating from carbon molecule's physical and chemical properties.

5 Conclusion/Summary

Millions of lives across the world have been affected by the COVID-19 pandemic, and everyone is still fighting to get through this stage of their lives together, and the whole world is trying to find a cure against this virus. Every person from different aspect of their life is trying to help the authority to tackle the infection. Doctors and healthcare officials are in the forefront of treating the COVID-19 infected individuals and social workers are at the forefront of ensuring that everybody gets the care and services they need, and researchers are trying to find a cure for this virus, and engineers are trying to build cost-effective ventilator systems and material researchers are trying to identify antiviral materials that can be used in masks and personal protective equipment. So now the fight against COVID is multidisciplinary, and in their own ways, everybody is trying to help. This chapter tried to summarize some of the simulation studies carried out to assess the efficacy of ventilation systems and the correct use of masks to minimize COVID-19 infection and also tried to integrate some of the studies already done in antiviral materials that can be used in masks and personal protective equipment.

Acknowledgements The author, Ms. Bhavya E V, acknowledges the Department of Science and Technology (DST), India for the financial support through INSPIRE Fellowship.

References

1. Mendez C, San José JF, Villafruela JM, Castro F (2008) Optimization of a hospital room by means of CFD for more efficient ventilation. Energy Build 40:849–854
2. Muia KW, Wonga LT, Wub CL, Lai Alvin CK (2009) Numerical modelling of exhaled droplet nuclei dispersion and mixing in indoor environments. J Hazard Mater 167:736–744
3. Zhao B et al (2009) How many airborne particles emitted from a nurse will reach the breathing zone/body surface of the patient in ISO Class-5 single-bed hospital protective environments? A numerical analysis. Aerosol Sci Technol 43(10):990–1005

4. Tunga YC, Hu SC, Tsaia TI, Changa IL (2009) An experimental study on ventilation efficiency of isolation room. Build Environ 44:271–279
5. Walker J, Hoffman P, Bennett A, Vos M, Thomas M, Tomlinson N (2007) Hospital and community acquired infection and the built environment—design and testing of infection control rooms. J Hosp Infect 65:43–49
6. Li Y, Leung GM, Tang JW, Yang X, Chao CY, Lin JZ, Lu JW (2007) Role of ventilation in airborne transmission of infectious agents in the built environment-a multidisciplinary systematic review. Indoor Air 17(1):2–18
7. Kermani A (2015) CFD modeling for ventilation system of a hospital room. In: Proceedings of the COMSOL Conference, vol 6
8. Mahajan P, Saco SA, Kumar RD, Raj RTK (2018) Airflow simulation of an isolation room using CFD technique. Int J Pure Appl Math 118(18):4261–4269
9. Balocco C (2011) Hospital ventilation simulation for the study of potential exposure to contaminants. Build Simul 4(1):5–20
10. Yu CP, Diu CK (1983) Total and regional deposition of inhaled aerosols in humans. J Aerosol Sci 14:599–609
11. Diekmann O, Heesterbeek JAP (2000) Mathematical epidemiology of infectious diseases. Wiley, Chichester, UK
12. Cunningham E (1910) On the velocity of steady fall of spherical particles through fluid medium. Proc R Soc Lond. A 83:357–365
13. Marianne T, Perini JM, Lafitte JJ, Houdret N, Pruvot FR, Lamblin G, Slayter HS, Roussel P (1987) Peptides of human bronchial mucus glycoproteins. Size determination by electron microscopy and by biosynthetic experiments. Biochem J 248:189–195
14. Tellier R (2006) Review of aerosol transmission of influenza a virus. Emerg Infect Dis 12 (11):1657
15. Batchelor CK, Batchelor G (2000) An introduction to fluid dynamics. Cambridge University Press
16. Jacob S, Yadav SS, Sikarwar BS (2019) Design and simulation of isolation room for a hospital. In: Advances in fluid and thermal engineering. Springer, pp 75–93
17. Jiang Y, Zhao B, Li X, Yang X, Zhang Z, Zhang Y (2009) Investigating a safe ventilation rate for the prevention of indoor SARS transmission: an attempt based on a simulation approach. Build Simul 2(4):281–289
18. Feng Y, Marchal T, Sperry T, Yi H (2020) Influence of wind and relative humidity on the social distancing effectiveness to prevent COVID-19 airborne transmission: a numerical study. J Aerosol Sci 105585
19. Lei Z, Yang J, Zhuang Z, Roberge R (2013) Simulation and evaluation of respirator faceseal leaks using computational fluid dynamics and infrared imaging. Ann Occup Hyg 57(4): 493–506
20. Lei Z, Yang J, Zhuang Z (2012) Headform and N95 filtering facepiece respirator interaction: contact pressure simulation and validation. J Occup Environ Hyg 9(1):46–58
21. Lei Z, Yang J, Zhuang Z (2010) Contact pressure study of N95 filtering face-piece respirators using finite element method. Comput-Aided Des Appl 7(6):847–861
22. De Greef S, Claes P, Vandermeulen D, Mollemans W, Suetens P, Willems G (2006) Large-scale in-vivo Caucasian facial soft tissue thickness database for craniofacial reconstruction. Forensic Sci Int 159:S126–S146
23. Oestenstad RK, Dillion HK, Perkins LL (1990) Distribution of faceseal leak sites on a half-mask respirator and their association with facial dimensions. Am Ind Hyg Assoc J 51:285–290
24. Oestenstad RK, Bartolucci AA (2010) Factors affecting the location and shape of face seal leak sites on half-mask respirators. J Occup Environ Hyg 7(6):332–341
25. Zhang X, Li H, Shen S, Rao Y, Chen F (2016) An improved FFR design with a ventilation fan: CFD simulation and validation. PloS ONE 11(7)
26. Zhou J, Hu Z, Zabihi F, Chen Z, Zhu M (2020) Progress and perspective of antiviral protective material. Adv Fiber Mater 1–17

27. Orlowski P et al (2018) Antiviral activity of tannic acid modified silver nanoparticles: potential to activate immune response in herpes genitalis. Viruses 10(10):524
28. Li Y, Lin Z, Zhao M, Xu T, Wang C, Hua L, Wang H, Xia H, Zhu B (2016) Silver nanoparticle based codelivery of oseltamivir to inhibit the activity of the H1N1 influenza virus through ROS-mediated signaling pathways. ACS Appl Mater Interfaces 8(37):24385–24393
29. Li Y et al (2016) Reversal of H1N1 influenza virus-induced apoptosis by silver nanoparticles functionalized with amantadine. RSC Adv 6(92):89679–89686
30. Lin Z et al (2017) The inhibition of H1N1 influenza virus-induced apoptosis by silver nanoparticles functionalized with zanamivir. RSC Adv 7(2):742–750
31. dos Santos Pereira AK et al (2019) Synthesis, crystallographic studies, molecular modeling and in vitro biological studies of silver (I) complexes with aminoadamantane ligands. Polyhedron 173:114116
32. Tang B, Li J, Hou X, Afrin T, Sun L, Wang X (2013) Colorful and antibacterial silk fiber from anisotropic silver nanoparticles. Ind Eng Chem Res 52(12):4556–4563
33. Jiang S, Qin W, Guo R, Zhang L (2010) Surface functionalization of nanostructured silver-coated polyester fabric by magnetron sputtering. Surf Coat Technol 204(21–22):3662–3667
34. Wu M, Ma B, Pan T, Chen S, Sun J (2016) Silver-nanoparticle-colored cotton fabrics with tunable colors and durable antibacterial and self-healing superhydrophobic properties. Adv Func Mater 26(4):569–576
35. Ali SW, Rajendran S, Joshi M (2011) Synthesis and characterization of chitosan and silver loaded chitosan nanoparticles for bioactive polyester. Carbohyd Polym 83(2):438–446
36. Li CM, Zheng LL, Yang XX, Wan XY, Wu WB, Zhen SJ, Li YF, Luo LF, Huang CZ (2016) DNA-AuNP networks on cell membranes as a protective barrier to inhibit viral attachment, entry and budding. Biomaterials 77:216–226
37. Bawage SS, Tiwari PM, Singh A, Dixit S, Pillai SR, Dennis VA, Singh SR (2016) Gold nanorods inhibit respiratory syncytial virus by stimulating the innate immune response. Nanomed: Nanotechnol Biol Med 12(8):2299–2310
38. Carja G, Grosu EF, Petrarean C, Nichita N (2015) Self-assemblies of plasmonic gold/layered double hydroxides with highly efficient antiviral effect against the hepatitis B virus. Nano Res 8(11):3512–3523
39. Zhou J, Xiang H, Zabihi F, Yu S, Sun B, Zhu M (2019) Intriguing anti-superbug Cu_2O@ ZrP hybrid nanosheet with enhanced antibacterial performance and weak cytotoxicity. Nano Res 12(6):1453–1460
40. Zhou J, Wang C, Cunningham AJ, Hu Z, Xiang H, Sun B, Zuo W, Zhu M (2019) Synthesis and characterization of size-controlled nano-Cu_2O deposited on alpha-zirconium phosphate with excellent antibacterial property. Mater Sci Eng, C 101:499–504
41. Borkow G, Zhou SS, Page T, Gabbay J (2010) A novel anti-influenza copper oxide containing respiratory face mask. PLoS One 5(6):e11295
42. Ye S, Shao K, Li Z, Guo N, Zuo Y, Li Q, Lu Z, Chen L, He Q, Han H (2015) Antiviral activity of graphene oxide: how sharp edged structure and charge matter. ACS Appl Mater Interfaces 7(38):21571–21579
43. Sametband M, Kalt I, Gedanken A, Sarid R (2014) Herpes simplex virus type-1 attachment inhibition by functionalized graphene oxide. ACS Appl Mater Interfaces 6(2):1228–1235

Chapter 10
A Detailed Scientometric Review of Coronavirus Research

A. K. Srivastava, Sarika Verma, Medha Mili, Samarendra Maji, Arfat Anis, S. A. R. Hashmi, and Kunal Pal

1 Introduction

In late December 2019, an emergence (COVID-19) was first diagnosed in Wuhan, China, occurring due to a novel coronavirus [1]. The coronavirus has now been rapidly spread to almost all parts of the world [2]. The global outbreak of the novel coronavirus disease or COVID-19 has been declared as a pandemic like Ebola, Zika, and Nipah by the World Health Organization (WHO) on March 12, 2020 [2]. This is now considered to be of major international concern toward public health. The coronavirus disease (COVID-19) is triggered by 2019-nCoV or most commonly known as severe acute respiratory syndrome coronavirus 2 (SARS-CoV-2), belonging to the β-coronavirus cluster [3].

Earlier, the world has witnessed an endemic situation in Guangdong, China (2002), due to a severe acute respiratory syndrome (SARS) outbreak that was caused by SARS-CoV [4]. After a decade in the year 2012, an endemic occurred in the Middle Eastern countries that were caused by Middle East respiratory syndrome

A. K. Srivastava · S. Verma (✉) · M. Mili · S. A. R. Hashmi
Council of Scientific and Industrial Research-Advanced Materials and Processes Research Institute (AMPRI), Hoshangabad Road, Bhopal, M.P 462026, India
e-mail: sarika.verma@ampri.res.in

S. Maji
Department of Chemistry, SRM Institute of Science and Technology, Kanchipuram, Tamil Nadu 603203, India

A. Anis
Department of Chemical Engineering, SABIC Polymer Research Center, King Saud University, Riyadh, Saudi Arabia

K. Pal (✉)
Department of Biotechnology and Medical Engineering, National Institute of Technology, Rourkela 769008, India
e-mail: palk@nitrkl.ac.in

M. Mohapatra et al. (eds.), *COVID-19 Pandemic*, Materials Horizons: From Nature to Nanomaterials, https://doi.org/10.1007/978-981-16-4372-9_10

coronavirus (MERS-CoV) [5]. Both the SARS-CoV and MERS-CoV belong to the β-coronavirus subgroup.

According to the report of the World Health Organization (WHO), the COVID-19 epidemic has already affected millions of people across the globe. The data itself is alarming, and the entire humanity is battling this era's most gut-wrenching war. However, till date, in the absence of specific therapeutic drugs or clinically approved vaccines for COVID-19, intensive research is urgently needed on the newly emerged SARS-CoV-2 to identify potential drug targets and for the eradication of the pathogenic mechanisms and epidemiological characteristics for the development of effective strategies for its prevention and treatment.

Coronaviruses (CoVs) consist of a single-stranded positive-sense RNA genome encapsulated within a membrane envelope [6, 7]. The coronaviruses consist of glycoprotein spikes on its outer surface, which are responsible for the attachment and entry of the virus to the host cells [8]. The receptor-binding domain (RBD) is loosely attached among the virus, which allows the virus to infect multiple hosts [9]. Their genomes contain 29,891 nucleotides that encode for 9860 amino acids [10]. CoVs are classified into four genera: Alphacoronavirus (alphaCoV), Betacoronavirus (betaCoV), Deltacoronavirus (deltaCoV), and Gammacoronavirus (gammaCoV) [11]. The SARS-CoV-2 belongs to the betaCoVs category and has a round, elliptic, or pleomorphic form, which has a diameter of 60–140 nm (approx.) [12, 13]. Similar to the other CoVs, they are sensitive to ultraviolet rays and heat. SARS-CoV-2 also possesses the typical coronavirus structure with spike protein [2]. This spike protein consists of a 3-D structure in the RBD region, which interacts with the host cells through the Van der Waals forces.

As reported in the literature, the SARS-CoV-2 also uses the same angiotensin-converting enzyme 2 (ACE2) cell receptor and the mechanism, which was previously used by the SARS-CoV for its entry into the host cell [7, 14]. SARS-CoV-2, similar to SARS-CoV and MERS-CoV, also attacks the lower respiratory system that causes viral pneumonia. Further, the virus also affects the gastrointestinal system, liver, kidney, heart, and central nervous system that lead to multiple organ failure [15].

According to recent information, SARS-CoV-2 is more transmissible/more contagious than SARS-CoV [7, 16]. A published report has revealed that the binding affinity of SARS-CoV-2 S protein to ACE2 is about 10−20 times higher than that of SARS-CoV S protein, which is speculated to be the reason behind the high transmissibility and contagiousness of SARS-CoV-2 as compared to SARS-CoV [7]. At the onset of the COVID-19, the main symptoms include fever, dry cough, fatigue, headache, and sore throat [17].

In severe cases, the patients may suffer from dyspnea and/or hypoxemia one week after the onset of the disease. But sometimes patients with even no obvious fever, mild fatigue, and no pneumonia, known as asymptomatic cases, can also spread SARS-CoV-2 between humans. The spread of the deadly virus from human-to-human is known to be transmitted via droplets or direct contact. Thus, there has been an urgent need for coronavirus-based research for detailed analysis in recent years. This will help in the availability of analyzed data under one common umbrella and thus will be helpful in future research work related to coronavirus. Unfortunately, there is no such scientometric review of the coronavirus-based research till now. A considerable amount of knowledge can be gained in a specific domain by having a systematic literature review in a relatively short time [18]. One of the quickest methods is the bibliometric analysis to perform literature review of a specific area for a large number of publications [18]. The bibliometric analysis supports us by providing the current trends in research of a specific field along with detailed understanding of the various relationship of author citation and author cooperation etc.

In view of the above discussions, we propose to introduce the bibliometric analysis of research based on coronavirus so as to gain an insight of the influential authors, institutions, and countries involved in the said research field, the most cited research articles and journals, and lastly, the recent trends in the field of the study. For the bibliometric analysis, the records of publications were retrieved from the database of Web of Science.

2 Methodology

2.1 *Data Source*

Publication information was obtained using the search engine of Web of Science (WOS) database, SCI-Expanded, which was deemed as the optimal database, was analyzed via bibliometric analysis.

2.2 *Search Strategy*

All the publication information was extracted from the Web of Science, and the database was collected on April 16, 2020. In our study, the research terms used for searching the articles were as follows: The database search was conducted using the parameters: TS = ((coronavirus) OR (coronavirus)). There was no restriction on the timespan, which resulted in the fetching of the documents from the year 2000 to 2020.

2.3 *Data Collection*

The total number of documents obtained was 11,925. From the obtained pool of publications, the document type was restricted to "Article," which reduced the count of publications to 9450. Further, the articles in "English" language were segregated. This process brought down the total number of documents to 9257. Then, the "full records with references" data of these publications were downloaded as.txt files with the Tab-delimited (Win, UTF-8) file format. The information on citations, bibliography, abstract and keywords, funding details, and all other information was exported as CSV files from the analyzed results of the Web of Science search engine.

2.4 Bibliometric and Visualized Analysis

The bibliometric analysis was performed using the VOS viewer software, developed by Van Eck and Waltman [19]. The intrinsic function of Web of Science was used to describe the essential features of the eligible desired publications network. These networks commonly include global researchers, journals, or individual publications and can be developed based on various factors like bibliographic couplings, citations, co-citations, authorship or co-authorship relationships, funding agencies, publication source, etc. The VOS viewer software creates a graphical representation of the bibliometric data [19]. The distances between the nodes within the graphical representation are related with the closeness between the nodes. Different bibliometric maps were generated and analyzed [18, 19].

3 Results and Discussions

3.1 Yearly Distribution and Trend of Growth

Altogether, a total 9257 number of articles were published on the topic related to coronavirus. This depicts that researchers and scientists had a great attraction and interest in this research field. The total count of publications that are published on year-on-year basis shows a good projection of the strength of research in a specific field. The analysis of the trends in the number of publications per year may divulge information on the research interest in the near future. A plot of the number of publications versus cumulative publications on a year-on-year basis was used to analyze the trend of research in the area of coronavirus in the past years (Fig. 1a). The analysis of the plot suggested that the research in the related field could be dated back to the year 2000. The highest number of publications (613 documents) was published in the year 2004. But in the year 2020, until now, i.e., 16 April 2020, 381 articles already had been published. The year 2002 has witnessed a very less number of publications (130 documents). Post-2002, there was an increase in the publications, which reached the maximum in the year 2004. This can be accounted for the fact that in late 2002, there was this SARS epidemic. Hence, there was a sudden increase in the field of coronavirus. However, post-2004, there was a

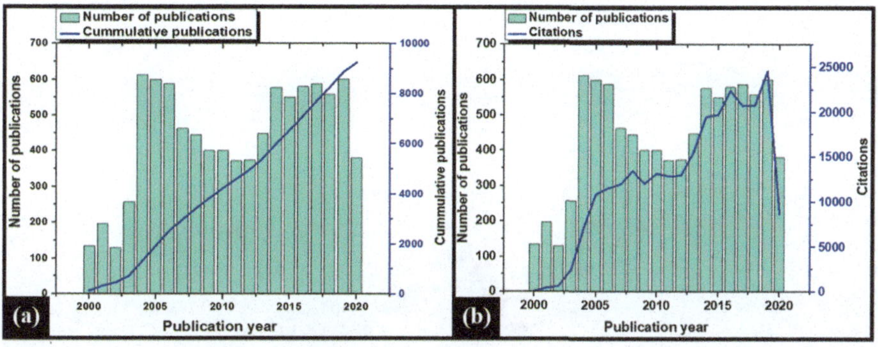

Fig. 1 Year-on-year publication information. **a** The number of publications and cumulative publications and **b** the number of publications and citations

decrease in the annual publications of articles until the year 2012. In late 2012, there was an outbreak of the Middle East respiratory syndrome (MERS). As a result of that, there was again an increase in the research in the field of coronavirus. Since the year 2014, the annual publications of the articles until the last year (2019) were similar. From the previous trends, it is quite expected that the number of publications is bound to increase in the year 2020. As a matter of fact, within the first three and a half months of the year 2020, nearly 400 articles on coronavirus have already been published. For the analysis of the graph of cumulative publications, the time period could be broadly divided into three main zones. The first zone of the period is between the years 2000 and 2004, wherein the research on coronavirus was increasing at a slow pace. Subsequently, during the period of 2004 to 2012, the momentum on the coronavirus research initially picked up. However, post-2006, the momentum was lost. In the third phase (2013–till date), there is a linear increase in coronavirus research. It is expected that the year 2020 will bring another turning point in coronavirus research across the globe.

The variation in the citations received by the publications during the 2000–2020 time periods has been summarized in Fig. 1b. During the period 2000 and 2002, the citations of the publications on coronavirus received very fewer citations. Since the year 2003, the number of citations had increased unexpectedly, and the increasing trend continued until 2008. This was quite expected because the researchers across the globe had started working on the coronavirus that was instigated by the SARS outbreak. Thereafter, until the year 2012, there was a plateau phase in terms of citations received by the publications on coronavirus. This suggested that the research on

coronavirus reached a stagnant phase. Since 2013, the number of citations per year showed an increasing trend even though the number of publications has remained fairly constant. This observation can be explained by the fact that the researchers were trying to gain insight on the coronavirus from the previously published publications. The average citation per year is 12,437. Although the year

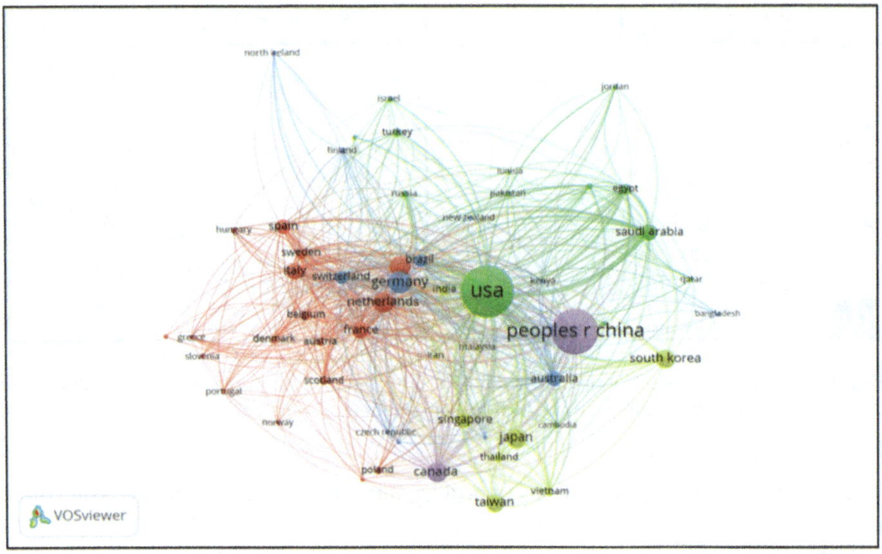

Fig. 2 Country cooperation network on coronavirus (N.B: (1) Countries that published at least more than ten documents were considered)

2020 has witnessed only just over 8500 citations, it is important to note that we are just within the first three and a half months of the year.

3.2 *Country-Level Distribution of Publications*

The 9257 number of documents was published from 126 countries, as tabulated in Table 1. The highest number of publications (3197 documents, 34.53% of the total documents) was reported from the United States of America (USA), followed by 2386 publications (25.77%) from Peoples R. China. Germany, the third rank holder, published 602 publications (6.50%). England and Netherlands were in fourth and fifth positions with 510 publications (5.50%) and 504 publications (5.44%), respectively. Further, the trend was followed by Japan, Canada, and South Korea. These countries had publications in the range of 406–470. Afterward, three countries that published documents were in the range of 329–366. Thereafter, five countries that published documents were in the range of 212–298, followed by another five countries that have published 115–189 documents. The analysis confirms the synergistic as well as a simultaneous approach between different countries in the area of coronavirus research. In total, 34 countries in the past had already published at least a hundred documents in the area of coronavirus. The statistics view of these countries is provided in Table 1. From the table, it is quite evident that 19 countries out of 56 countries had a nominal GDP rank below 20 indicating that

Table 1 Top countries that published more than ten documents

#	Country	Documents	% of 9257	Citations	Average citations per documents	Nominal GDP rank[a]	Total link strength
1	USA	3184	34.536	110,117	34.58	1	1941
2	Peoples R China	2382	25.775	65,472	27.49	2	1123
3	Germany	598	6.503	28,688	47.97	4	799
4	Netherlands	504	5.509	30,408	60.33	17	626
5	England	500	5.445	17,734	35.47	7	697
6	Japan	470	5.088	8794	18.71	3	196
7	Canada	461	5.002	17,417	37.78	10	407
8	South Korea	406	4.407	6934	17.08	12	152
9	Taiwan	366	3.954	9715	26.54	22	111
10	France	352	3.824	11,987	34.05	6	534
11	Italy	329	3.554	7234	21.99	8	276
12	Saudi Arabia	298	3.219	11,100	37.25	19	413
13	Singapore	277	3.003	10,557	38.11	38	229
14	Australia	274	2.982	9820	35.84	14	324
15	Spain	234	2.528	6979	29.82	13	226
16	Switzerland	212	2.301	9697	45.74	20	411
17	Brazil	189	2.042	1917	10.14	9	89
18	Sweden	133	1.437	4555	34.25	24	206
19	Belgium	122	1.329	2858	23.43	25	129
20	Egypt	117	1.264	2149	18.37	40	230
21	India	115	1.264	1637	14.23	5	84
22	Scotland	87	0.961	3710	42.64	–	166
23	Thailand	86	0.929	4016	46.70	23	90
24	Turkey	78	0.843	977	12.53	18	38
25	Poland	67	0.724	785	11.72	21	63
26	Austria	59	0.648	2550	43.22	28	96
27	Denmark	59	0.637	1408	23.86	39	107
28	Vietnam	59	0.637	2863	48.53	44	123
29	United Arab Emirates	54	0.583	1257	23.28	31	85
30	Finland	49	0.529	2626	53.59	45	55
31	South Africa	48	0.519	1279	26.65	37	70
32	Russia	47	0.508	1381	29.38	11	74
33	Iran	42	0.465	278	6.62	27	15

(continued)

Table 1 (continued)

#	Country	Documents	% of 9257	Citations	Average citations per documents	Nominal GDP rank[a]	Total link strength
34	Hungary	41	0.443	872	21.27	–	49
35	Israel	35	0.378	810	23.14	32	29
36	Mexico	32	0.346	1127	35.22	15	49
37	Kenya	31	0.335	1060	34.19	–	76
38	Malaysia	31	0.335	278	8.97	36	27
39	Norway	31	0.335	781	25.19	30	24
40	Greece	29	0.313	413	14.24	–	56
41	Portugal	24	0.259	377	15.71	49	41
42	Argentina	23	0.259	491	21.35	29	19
43	Qatar	23	0.248	732	31.83	–	36
44	Jordan	22	0.248	568	25.82	–	36
45	Czech Republic	18	0.216	628	34.89	–	29
46	Ireland	18	0.194	413	22.94	33	33
47	New Zealand	18	0.194	917	50.94	–	13
48	Pakistan	18	0.194	310	17.22	48	32
49	North Ireland	15	0.184	1085	72.33	–	29
50	Slovenia	15	0.162	297	19.80	–	21
51	Bangladesh	14	0.151	485	34.64	–	17
52	Tunisia	14	0.151	226	16.14	–	23
53	Ghana	13	0.14	608	46.77	–	33
54	Nigeria	13	0.14	418	32.15	26	34
55	Cambodia	12	0.13	210	17.50	–	45
56	Croatia	10	0.108	72	7.20	–	10

[a]Nominal GDP Rank as per the International Monetary Fund (2020 estimates), World Economic Outlook Database, February 2020

the economically developed countries are carrying out research on coronavirus. The USA has the most number of 110,117 citations from the 3184 documents, followed by Peoples R. China, Netherlands, Germany, and England. The publications from these countries had received 65,472, 30,408, 28,688, and 17,734 citations, respectively. Interestingly, the average citation per documents of North Ireland was in the first position (72.33) from 15 documents, followed by the Netherlands with an average citation of 60.33 from a total of 604 documents. Germany, England, Finland, and New Zealand, respectively, were subsequently in order of the countries that had an average citation of 50 or higher. It is important to note that India is ranked twenty-first, in terms of the published number of documents with an average citation per document of 14.23.

According to the VOS viewer manual, each and every link is assigned a strength, which is shown by a positive numerical value. The higher the value, the stronger is the link. In other words, the link and the assigned strength are directly proportional to each other. The TLS highlights the total number of publications with at least a common two keywords in the documents. The TLS also gives information related to the collaborative research in the common research area among different countries. The analysis of TLS, as shown in Table 1, suggested that USA, had TLS of 1941, was the most superior country by far in terms of collaborative research. USA was the major contributor in the area of coronavirus research and globally played a leading role. It was found that the USA had documents published in collaboration with many countries like Argentina, Cambodia, Egypt, Israel, Jordan, Nigeria, Pakistan, Qatar, Russia, Saudi Arabia, Tunisia, Turkey, and United Arab Emirates (Fig. 2). China was in the second position, with a TLS of 1123, followed by Germany in the third position with a TLS score of 799 in the collaborative research. The TLS score along with the cooperation network map suggests a strong research collaboration of many countries with USA and China. In the fourth and fifth positions were England and Netherlands, with a TLS of 626 and 697, respectively.

3.3 *The Co-Authorship and Organizations Relationship*

Further, the co-authorship and organization relationship was studied with a minimum number of documents of an organization and citations of an organization of being 10 and 1000 in number, respectively. Accordingly, the data of 150 organizations was obtained and is presented in Fig. 3 and Table 2. It shows that the University of Hong Kong was in the first position with 417 documents and 56.62 average citations. The TLS of the University of Hong Kong was 384. After the University of Hong Kong, the Chinese Academy of Science with 306 documents, 33.80 average citations, and 283 TLS was in the second position. The third position was occupied by the "Center for Disease Control and Prevention," which have 191 documents, 55.87 average citations per document, and TLS of 210. Univ Utrecht and Chinese Academy Gramsci have 184 and 162 documents with 45.80 and 17.41 average citations and 170 and 45 TLS with other organizations.

3.4 *Relationship of Authors and Co-Authors*

The author and co-authorship network visualization map was created on the basis of bibliographic data gathered from the core collection. The analysis helps in identifying the major groups across the globe that is working in a research field related to coronavirus. This is achieved easily by mapping the relationship of authors with the co-author, as depicted in Table S2 and Fig. 4, respectively. Easy and visual representation of the relationship is obtained using the mapping process, which makes

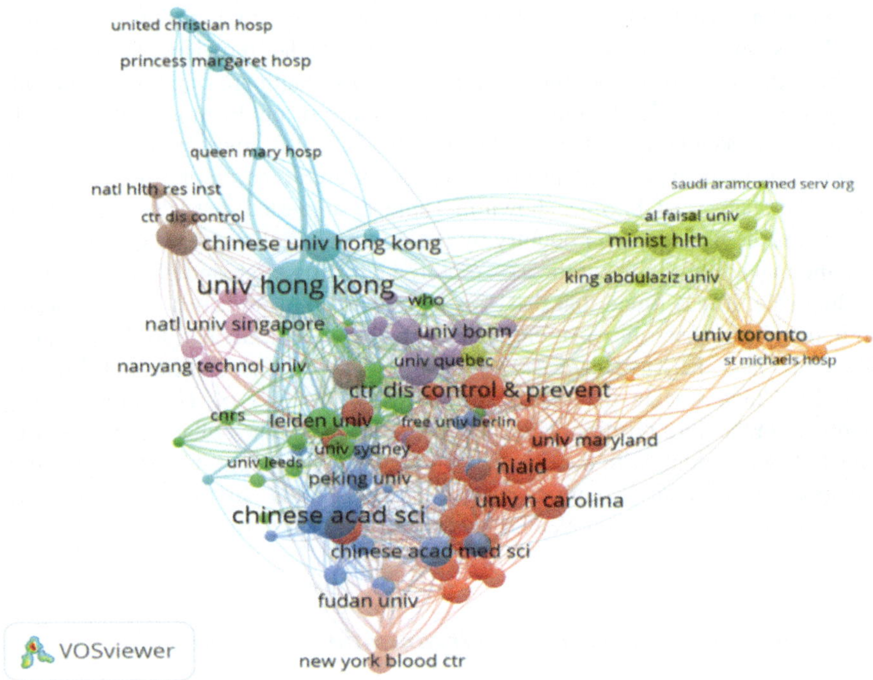

Fig. 3 Co-authorship—organizations of the researchers who are working in the area of coronavirus research. (N.B.: (1) Authors who have published at least ten documents were considered)

the study of both the individual activity of an author as well its interconnectivity with other research groups much easier. Figure 5 depicts five major groups (considering the presence of at least five authors in each group) that are working in the field of coronavirus. The research group of the author named Yuen Kwok-yung was the prominent group in the research field of coronavirus. Yuen Kwok-yung had the highest number of documents (number of documents = 120) among all other researchers, followed by Ralph S. Baric and Christian Drosten, with 111 and 109 total number of documents, respectively. The analysis of the TLS suggests that there is a significant research collaboration work among many of the researchers. However, some of the researchers are not involved in much research collaboration. It is of understanding that research collaboration improves critical information and knowledge flow among the different research groups all over the world. Extensive research collaboration among all the authors will definitely help in enhancing the improvement in the quality of the research on coronavirus. Further, Table 3 depicts the details of the count of published documents by the authors and their citation metrics, which helps to identify the most active researchers in this coronavirus research field. As already mentioned, the authors Kwok-Yung Yuen, Ralph S.Baric, and Christian Drosten had the highest number of published documents. However,

Table 2 Co-authorship and organizations relationship

Id	Organization	Documents	Citations	Average citations per document	TLS
1	Univ Hong Kong	417	23,612	56.62	384
2	Chinese Acad Sci	306	10,342	33.80	283
3	Ctr Dis Control and Prevent	191	10,672	55.87	210
4	Univ Utrecht	184	8427	45.80	170
5	Chinese Acad Agr Sci	162	2821	17.41	45
6	Chinese Univ Hong Kong	162	5209	32.15	124
7	Univ N Carolina	155	6759	43.61	153
8	Niaid	149	7380	49.53	181
9	Univ Iowa	140	4257	30.41	98
10	Univ Penn	132	4395	33.30	100
11	Leiden Univ	124	7179	57.90	119
12	Natl Inst Infect Dis	124	2413	19.46	21
13	Chinese Acad Med Sci	121	3760	31.07	212
14	Minist Hlth	115	5307	46.15	285
15	Natl Taiwan Univ	114	2698	23.67	86
16	Fudan Univ	109	2858	26.22	193
17	Seoul Natl Univ	109	2451	22.49	11
18	Univ Bonn	104	6108	58.73	165
19	Erasmus Mc	101	7146	70.75	105
20	Univ Calif Davis	100	2749	27.49	59
21	Ohio State Univ	98	2665	27.19	46
22	Univ Toronto	98	4641	47.36	208
23	Acad Sinica	97	2799	28.86	102
24	Natl Univ Singapore	92	3695	40.16	63
25	Vanderbilt Univ	92	4215	45.82	89
26	Univ Georgia	88	1895	21.53	51
27	Univ Minnesota	88	2343	26.63	101
28	Csic	87	2862	32.90	28
29	Peking Union Med Coll	85	2646	31.13	176
30	Univ Washington	83	3699	44.57	111
31	Peking Univ	81	2087	25.77	53
32	Cornell Univ	78	2430	31.15	51
33	Inst Pasteur	78	4386	56.23	111
34	Scripps Res Inst	78	3007	38.55	81
35	Johns Hopkins Univ	76	2374	31.24	58
36	Sun Yat Sen Univ	76	1286	16.92	61
37	Harvard Univ	75	5997	79.96	88
38	New York Blood Ctr	74	2591	35.01	155
39	Univ Oxford	74	2484	33.57	147

(continued)

Table 2 (continued)

Id	Organization	Documents	Citations	Average citations per document	TLS
40	Nanyang Technol Univ	71	1553	21.87	51
41	Wuhan Univ	69	1821	26.39	58
42	Univ Illinois	67	1700	25.37	57
43	Chinese Ctr Dis Control and Prevent	66	1815	27.50	99
44	Univ Colorado	65	2109	32.45	50
45	Univ Maryland	65	2074	31.91	53
46	Univ Texas Med Branch	65	1702	26.18	86
47	Natl Yang Ming Univ	63	1336	21.21	40
48	Purdue Univ	62	1478	23.84	42
49	Univ So Calif	62	2329	37.56	25
50	Zhejiang Univ	62	1680	27.10	61
51	King Saud Univ	60	1233	20.55	114
52	Tsinghua Univ	59	1641	27.81	55
53	Acad Mil Med Sci	58	1116	19.24	55
54	Beijing Inst Microbiol and Epidemiol	58	1768	30.48	122
55	Univ Tennessee	58	1311	22.60	31
56	Loyola Univ	56	2755	49.20	63
57	Univ Amsterdam	54	2398	44.41	43
58	Univ Zurich	54	2793	51.72	68
59	Inst Mol and Cell Biol	53	1493	28.17	40
60	Texas A & M Univ	53	1336	25.21	18
61	Univ Calif Irvine	51	1736	34.04	38
62	Iowa State Univ	50	1739	34.78	36
63	Univ Sydney	50	1322	26.44	41
64	Washington Univ	49	3176	64.82	68
65	Columbia Univ	48	2235	46.56	61
66	Nih	48	2922	60.88	92
67	Princess Margaret Hosp	48	3164	65.92	70
68	Alfaisal Univ	47	1516	32.26	163
69	Kansas State Univ	47	1010	21.49	42
70	Univ Calif San Francisco	46	5977	129.93	56
71	Shanghai Jiao Tong Univ	45	1261	28.02	49
72	Univ Florida	45	1087	24.16	55
73	Univ Texas	45	2472	54.93	22
74	Univ Wurzburg	44	4309	97.93	50
75	Univ Manitoba	42	2348	55.90	38
76	Singapore Gen Hosp	41	3392	82.73	50
77	Univ Bristol	41	1396	34.05	60

(continued)

Table 2 (continued)

Id	Organization	Documents	Citations	Average citations per document	TLS
78	Univ Quebec	41	1242	30.29	15
79	Emory Univ	40	1677	41.93	73
80	King Faisal Specialist Hosp and Res Ctr	40	1548	38.70	105
81	Natl Hlth Res Inst	40	1167	29.18	46
82	Ucl	40	3497	87.43	131
83	Univ Edinburgh	40	2271	56.78	78
84	Who	40	3173	79.33	77
85	Natl Vet Inst	39	1390	35.64	17
86	Cnrs	36	1759	48.86	68
87	Colorado State Univ	36	1301	36.14	42
88	King Abdulaziz Univ	36	1531	42.53	70
89	Mt Sinai Hosp	36	2380	66.11	89
90	Univ British Columbia	36	3556	98.78	38
91	Ecohlth Alliance	34	1637	48.15	56
92	Indiana Univ Sch Med	34	1623	47.74	108
93	New York State Dept Hlth	34	1940	57.06	26
94	Tan Tock Seng Hosp	34	1127	33.15	42
95	Nci	33	1292	39.15	34
96	Robert Koch Inst	33	1563	47.36	47
97	Univ Med Ctr Utrecht	33	1686	51.09	35
98	Univ Reading	33	1292	39.15	41
99	Cleveland Clin	32	1420	44.38	47
100	Ctr Dis Control	32	4192	131.00	44
101	Univ Virginia	32	1099	34.34	92
102	Mcmaster Univ	31	1330	42.90	49
103	Bernhard Nocht Inst Trop Med	30	5148	171.60	54
104	United Christian Hosp	30	2829	94.30	56
105	Univ Giessen	30	1389	46.30	41
106	Univ Leeds	30	1059	35.30	15
107	Univ London Imperial Coll Sci Technol and Med	30	1556	51.87	40
108	Univ Helsinki	29	1099	37.90	23
109	Free Univ Berlin	28	1048	37.43	28
110	Inst Anim Hlth	28	1404	50.14	8
111	Karolinska Inst	28	1996	71.29	50
112	Yale Univ	28	1071	38.25	17
113	Usda Ars	27	1230	45.56	19
114	Queen Mary Hosp	26	3273	125.88	46

(continued)

Table 2 (continued)

Id	Organization	Documents	Citations	Average citations per document	TLS
115	Univ Queensland	26	1499	57.65	24
116	Beijing Inst Radiat Med	25	1240	49.60	22
117	Natl Inst Publ Hlth and Environm	25	1539	61.56	35
118	Univ Hlth Network	23	1529	66.48	55
119	Univ Marburg	23	2934	127.57	27
120	Univ Massachusetts	23	1928	83.83	29
121	Pamela Youde Nethersole Eastern Hosp	22	2468	112.18	30
122	Tsing Hua Univ	22	1014	46.09	24
123	Univ Hosp	22	1110	50.45	11
124	Al Faisal Univ	21	2377	113.19	77
125	Kantonal Hosp St Gallen	21	1730	82.38	51
126	King Abdul Aziz Med City	20	1006	50.30	60
127	Csiro Livestock Ind	19	1544	81.26	13
128	Gordon Life Sci Inst	19	1484	78.11	18
129	Prince Sultan Mil Med City	19	1406	74.00	97
130	Univ Freiburg	19	1638	86.21	36
131	Guangzhou Ctr Dis Control and Prevent	18	1700	94.44	24
132	USA	18	1504	83.56	29
133	Dept Hlth	16	3069	191.81	36
134	Hosp Sick Children	16	1630	101.88	44
135	Univ Aix Marseille 1	16	1044	65.25	43
136	Univ Aix Marseille 2	16	1044	65.25	43
137	Goethe Univ Frankfurt	15	2999	199.93	18
138	Mt Sinai Sch Med	14	1383	98.79	20
139	Tufts Univ	14	1272	90.86	9
140	Hlth Protect Agcy	13	1096	84.31	20
141	Saudi Aramco Med Serv Org	13	1804	138.77	60
142	St Michaels Hosp	13	1510	116.15	42
143	Karolinska Univ Hosp	12	1629	135.75	19
144	Queen Elizabeth Hosp	12	2285	190.42	27
145	Erasmus Univ	11	3557	323.36	15
146	Royal Childrens Hosp	11	1255	114.09	13
147	Wellcome Trust Sanger Inst	11	1300	118.18	50
148	Austrian Acad Sci	10	1228	122.80	23
149	Erasmus Med Ctr	10	1952	195.20	16
150	Toronto Med Labs	10	1118	111.80	33

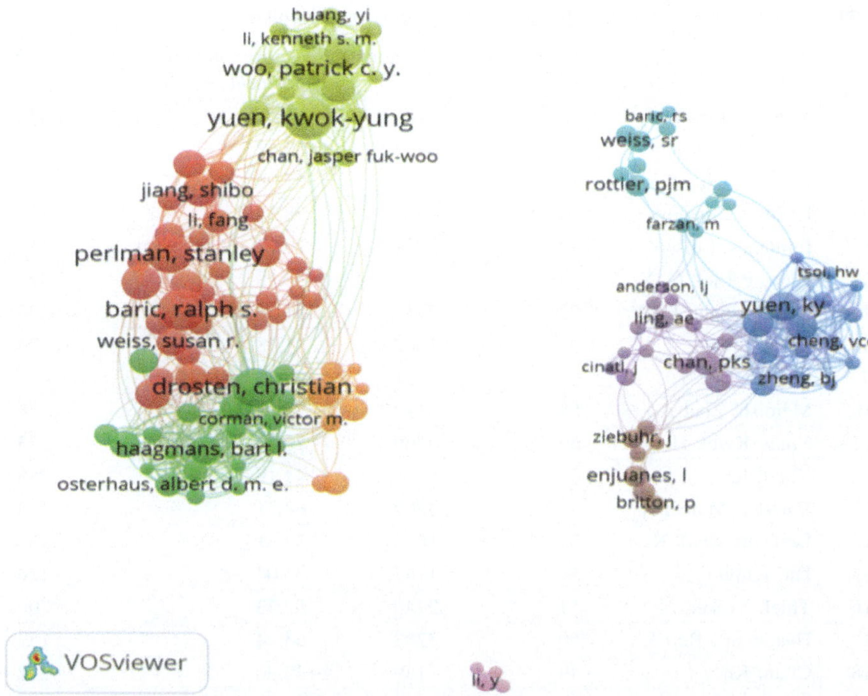

Fig. 4 Authors and co-authors relationship of the researchers who are working in the area of coronavirus research (N.B.: (1) Authors who have published at least twenty-five documents were considered)

the highest number of citations is of Ky Yuen, followed by Khandyuen Chan and Kwok-Yung Yuen, respectively, which indicated that these three authors are the most cited researchers on coronavirus across the globe. However, the information about the most impactful researchers can be provided by the average citations per document. In other words, a good quality paper can be identified by calculating average citations per document. It was found that W. Lim (documents: 14 citations: 411) followed by Lj Anderson (documents: 10 citations: 396), Adme Osterhaus (documents: 16 citations: 344), Ron A. M. Fouchier (documents: 11, citations: 245) and Theo M. Bestebroer (documents: 10, citations: 233) had the highest average citations per document. This is suggestive of the fact that the documents of W. Lim, Lj Anderson, Adme Osterhaus, Lj, Ron A. M. Fouchier and Theo M.Bestebroer were more impactful as compared to the others.

Table 3 Top authors who published more than twenty-five documents

Id	Author	Documents	Citations	Average citations per document	TLS
1	Yuen, Kwok-Yung	120	6176	51.47	420
2	Baric, Ralph S	111	3843	34.62	86
3	Drosten, Christian	104	5614	53.98	250
4	Perlman, Stanley	99	2790	28.18	86
5	Enjuanes, Luis	77	2251	29.23	51
6	Woo, Patrick C. Y	74	3935	53.18	325
7	Lau, Susanna K. P	72	3714	51.58	324
8	Jiang, Shibo	63	2002	31.78	125
9	Snijder, Eric J	63	3131	49.70	42
10	Memish, Ziad A	58	4198	72.38	118
11	Chan, Kwok-Hung	56	4269	76.23	253
12	Yuen, Ky	56	8074	144.18	255
13	Mueller, Marcel A	53	3297	62.21	160
14	Denison, Mark R	51	1663	32.61	36
15	Du, Lanying	51	1787	35.04	126
16	Thiel, Volker	51	2740	53.73	70
17	Haagmans, Bart L	50	3287	65.74	152
18	Chan, Kh	49	7149	145.90	242
19	Weiss, Susan R	49	1141	23.29	11
20	Peiris, Jsm	48	7789	162.27	200
21	Rottier, Peter J. M	47	2128	45.28	63
22	Zheng, Bo-Jian	45	2548	56.62	149
23	Saif, Linda J	41	1077	26.27	2
24	Wang, Lin-Fa	41	1499	36.56	18
25	Zhao, Jincun	41	1332	32.49	48
26	Baker, Susan C	40	1656	41.40	11
27	Chan, Pks	40	2208	55.20	51
28	Li, Fang	38	1136	29.89	49
29	Al-Tawfiq, Jaffar A	37	2516	68.00	72
30	Osterhaus, Albert D. M. E	35	3788	108.23	92
31	Zhou, Yusen	35	1046	29.89	100
32	Gerber, Susan I	34	1049	30.85	11
33	Guan, Y	34	7414	218.06	152
34	Sung, Jjy	33	1561	47.30	45
35	Frieman, Matthew B	32	1306	40.81	17
36	Rottier, Pjm	32	2350	73.44	25
37	Graham, Rachel L	31	1130	36.45	43
38	De Haan, Cornelis A. M	30	1052	35.07	35

(continued)

Table 3 (continued)

Id	Author	Documents	Citations	Average citations per document	TLS
39	Drexler, Jan Felix	30	1399	46.63	64
40	Gorbalenya, Alexander E	30	1535	51.17	34
41	Poon, Llm	30	6923	230.77	138
42	Weiss, Sr	30	1040	34.67	14
43	Ziebuhr, John	30	1004	33.47	19
44	Enjuanes, L	29	1601	55.21	2
45	Raj, V. Stalin	29	2700	93.10	117
46	Bosch, Berend-Jan	28	1485	53.04	65
47	Dijkman, Ronald	28	1290	46.07	52
48	Tseng, Chien-Te K	27	1147	42.48	41
49	Cavanagh, D	26	1357	52.19	25
50	Katze, Michael G	26	1198	46.08	32
51	Dediego, Marta L	25	1034	41.36	37
52	Gao, George F	25	1320	52.80	11
53	Li, Y	25	2633	105.32	19

3.5 *Relationship of Distribution and Co-Citation*

The relationship between sources and citations helps in concluding the interest of authors in which journals they prefer to publish their research results. The research articles that had published related to coronavirus in the important journals in the last twenty years are depicted in Table 4 and Fig. 5, respectively. From Table 4, it can be concluded that the most preferred and accepted choice is the "Journal of Virology" of many authors to publish their coronavirus-related research work. In the journal, till date 886 numbers of documents have been published with gathering 39,407 citations for the journal. The Journal "Virology" occupied the second position where 285 numbers of documents have been published with 7759 citations followed by the journal "PlOS One," in the third position where 341 publications were published and had received 4488 citations for these articles. The aforesaid three journals had a good TLS, suggesting that these journals were highly cited. This observation can also be confirmed from the source-citation relationship map. The average citations per document provide an indication of the impactful publications that are published in the journals. Taking into account the average citations per documents, the top journals were The New England Journal of Medicine and Science with 15 documents, each with 530.27 and 419.90 average citations per document. Nature Medicine has 13 documents with 178.15 average citations per document. Also, the journals proceedings of the National Academy of Sciences of the United States of America have 111 documents but have105 average citations per document. Similarly, The Lancet Infectious Diseases has only 36 and

Table 4 Top Journals where more than ten documents were published

Id	Source	Documents	Citations	Average Citations Per Document	TLS
1	Journal Of Virology	886	39,407	44.48	21,327
2	Virology	285	7759	27.22	7231
3	Plos One	241	4488	18.62	3795
4	Emerging Infectious Diseases	203	9300	45.81	4559
5	Journal Of General Virology	188	5877	31.26	4567
6	Virus Research	175	3251	18.58	4782
7	Archives Of Virology	159	2693	16.94	2395
8	Journal Of Virological Methods	149	2783	18.68	1867
9	Veterinary Microbiology	146	2706	18.53	2145
10	Journal Of Medical Virology	131	4159	31.75	1754
11	Viruses-Basel	115	916	7.97	2357
12	Journal Of Clinical Microbiology	112	5542	49.48	1947
13	Proceedings Of The National Academy Of Sciences Of The United States Of America	111	11,439	103.05	5364
14	Vaccine	99	2190	22.12	1926
15	Virology Journal	97	1611	16.61	1638
16	Antiviral Research	96	1709	17.80	1634
17	Journal Of Clinical Virology	93	2760	29.68	1357
18	Journal Of Infectious Diseases	93	4012	43.14	2185
19	Avian Diseases	92	1993	21.66	1016
20	Biochemical And Biophysical Research Communications	92	3366	36.59	2089
21	Virus Genes	92	1849	20.10	1576
22	Nidoviruses: Toward Control Of Sars And Other Nidovirus Diseases	89	369	4.15	889
23	Plos Pathogens	85	4610	54.24	2742
24	Scientific Reports	81	876	10.81	1377
25	Journal Of Biological Chemistry	79	4255	53.86	2520
26	Eurosurveillance	68	1975	29.04	1071
27	Clinical Infectious Diseases	64	4566	71.34	1235
28	Nidoviruses (Coronaviruses And Arteriviruses)	63	282	4.48	200
29	Journal Of Feline Medicine And Surgery	61	1018	16.69	584
30	Journal Of Veterinary Diagnostic Investigation	60	1436	23.93	642

(continued)

Table 4 (continued)

Id	Source	Documents	Citations	Average Citations Per Document	TLS
31	Mbio	57	2709	47.53	2104
32	Avian Pathology	56	1588	28.36	1109
33	BMC Infectious Diseases	56	1067	19.05	638
34	Journal Of Veterinary Medical Science	56	525	9.38	448
35	Infection Genetics And Evolution	55	847	15.40	1136
36	Journal Of Immunology	55	2526	45.93	1095
37	Emerging Microbes and Infections	46	372	8.09	1027
38	Transboundary And Emerging Diseases	45	541	12.02	646
39	BMC Veterinary Research	41	410	10.00	459
40	Pediatric Infectious Disease Journal	41	1413	34.46	459
41	Febs Letters	40	1100	27.50	898
42	Journal Of Wildlife Diseases	39	654	16.77	108
43	Current Opinion In Virology	37	855	23.11	970
44	Influenza And Other Respiratory Viruses	36	489	13.58	295
45	Lancet	36	8666	240.72	3005
46	Viral Immunology	35	360	10.29	444
47	International Journal Of Infectious Diseases	34	877	25.79	501
48	Nucleic Acids Research	34	1360	40.00	403
49	Veterinary Record	32	711	22.22	288
50	Chinese Medical Journal	31	218	7.03	324
51	Research In Veterinary Science	31	312	10.06	326
52	Bioorganic and Medicinal Chemistry	30	574	19.13	450
53	Bioorganic and Medicinal Chemistry Letters	30	677	22.57	347
54	Veterinary Immunology And Immunopathology	30	595	19.83	319
55	Journal Of Medicinal Chemistry	29	1061	36.59	566
56	Journal Of Molecular Biology	29	1651	56.93	1229
57	Veterinary Journal	28	568	20.29	274
58	Biochemistry	27	794	29.41	744
59	Clinical And Vaccine Immunology	27	287	10.63	345

(continued)

Table 4 (continued)

Id	Source	Documents	Citations	Average Citations Per Document	TLS
60	Epidemiology And Infection	27	199	7.37	255
61	Veterinary Research	26	264	10.15	433
62	Clinical And Diagnostic Laboratory Immunology	25	528	21.12	443
63	Poultry Science	25	252	10.08	252
64	American Journal Of Infection Control	23	210	9.13	156
65	Japanese Journal Of Infectious Diseases	23	160	6.96	222
66	Preventive Veterinary Medicine	22	436	19.82	190
67	Journal Of Infection And Public Health	21	128	6.10	203
68	Microbes And Infection	21	270	12.86	404
69	Acta Crystallographica Section F-Structural Biology Communications	20	65	3.25	219
70	Antiviral Therapy	20	417	20.85	249
71	Intervirology	19	130	6.84	270
72	Journal Of Infection	19	615	32.37	276
73	Journal Of Infection In Developing Countries	19	94	4.95	180
74	Journal Of Korean Medical Science	19	158	8.32	117
75	Nature	19	4823	253.84	1729
76	Pediatrics	19	1040	54.74	246
77	Zoonoses And Public Health	19	242	12.74	249
78	Frontiers In Microbiology	18	100	5.56	296
79	Journal Of Veterinary Internal Medicine	18	303	16.83	151
80	Acta Veterinaria Hungarica	17	78	4.59	79
81	Antimicrobial Agents And Chemotherapy	17	637	37.47	347
82	Chest	17	748	44.00	155
83	Clinical Microbiology And Infection	17	493	29.00	218
84	Journal Of Comparative Pathology	17	272	16.00	179
85	Acta Virologica	16	98	6.13	155
86	American Journal Of Pathology	16	629	39.31	314
87	American Journal Of Veterinary Research	16	287	17.94	175

(continued)

Table 4 (continued)

Id	Source	Documents	Citations	Average Citations Per Document	TLS
88	Journal Of Hospital Infection	16	333	20.81	189
89	Journal Of Neurovirology	16	206	12.88	144
90	Journal Of Theoretical Biology	16	676	42.25	80
91	Lancet Infectious Diseases	16	1897	118.56	934
92	Veterinary Pathology	16	304	19.00	215
93	Canadian Journal Of Veterinary Research-Revue Canadienne De Recherche Veterinaire	15	246	16.40	105
94	Chinese Science Bulletin	15	127	8.47	129
95	European Journal Of Clinical Microbiology and Infectious Diseases	15	166	11.07	167
96	European Journal Of Medicinal Chemistry	15	334	22.27	134
97	Journal Of Neuroimmunology	15	141	9.40	106
98	Nature Communications	15	464	30.93	446
99	New England Journal Of Medicine	15	7954	530.27	3591
100	Respirology	15	351	23.40	145
101	Science	15	6294	419.60	2992
102	Journal Of Microbiology And Biotechnology	14	65	4.64	132
103	Virologica Sinica	14	107	7.64	276
104	Acta Crystallographica Section D-Structural Biology	13	117	9.00	250
105	Diagnostic Microbiology And Infectious Disease	13	177	13.62	146
106	Infection Control And Hospital Epidemiology	13	165	12.69	83
107	Nature Medicine	13	2316	178.15	904
108	Australian Veterinary Journal	12	219	18.25	153
109	BMC Bioinformatics	12	256	21.33	100
110	BMC Genomics	12	238	19.83	140
111	Clinical Chemistry	12	472	39.33	261
112	DNA And Cell Biology	12	157	13.08	171
113	Immunology	12	283	23.58	132
114	Journal Of Biomedical Science	12	171	14.25	253
115	Microbiology And Immunology	12	79	6.58	233
116	Molecular And Cellular Probes	12	166	13.83	99

(continued)

Table 4 (continued)

Id	Source	Documents	Citations	Average Citations Per Document	TLS
117	Msphere	12	55	4.58	131
118	Protein Science	12	248	20.67	274
119	Proteomics	12	348	29.00	200
120	Tropical Animal Health And Production	12	91	7.58	89
121	Vector-Borne And Zoonotic Diseases	12	163	13.58	138
122	Acta Veterinaria Scandinavica	11	164	14.91	76
123	Applied Microbiology And Biotechnology	11	105	9.55	111
124	Brazilian Journal Of Microbiology	11	26	2.36	57
125	Cell Research	11	542	49.27	392
126	Cellular Microbiology	11	367	33.36	212
127	Comparative Medicine	11	137	12.45	41
128	Febs Journal	11	210	19.09	180
129	Infectious Disease Clinics Of North America	11	158	14.36	294
130	Journal Of The Formosan Medical Association	11	124	11.27	67
131	Journal Of Veterinary Medicine Series B-Infectious Diseases And Veterinary Public Health	11	516	46.91	92
132	Journal Of Veterinary Science	11	80	7.27	114
133	Journal Of Zoo And Wildlife Medicine	11	150	13.64	33
134	Molecular Immunology	11	142	12.91	184
135	Revue Scientifique Et Technique-Office International Des Epizooties	11	44	4.00	155
136	Structure	11	738	67.09	282
137	Travel Medicine And Infectious Disease	11	134	12.18	143
138	American Journal Of Respiratory And Critical Care Medicine	10	641	64.10	155
139	Biochemical Journal	10	244	24.40	158
140	Bioinformatics	10	183	18.30	43
141	Biomedical And Environmental Sciences	10	90	9.00	76

(continued)

Table 4 (continued)

Id	Source	Documents	Citations	Average Citations Per Document	TLS
142	Cell Host and Microbe	10	754	75.40	333
143	Ecohealth	10	167	16.70	106
144	Frontiers In Immunology	10	119	11.90	116
145	Human Vaccines and Immunotherapeutics	10	95	9.50	198
146	Journal Of Dairy Science	10	282	28.20	51
147	Protein Expression And Purification	10	124	12.40	110
148	Scandinavian Journal Of Infectious Diseases	10	146	14.60	97
149	Thorax	10	610	61.00	146

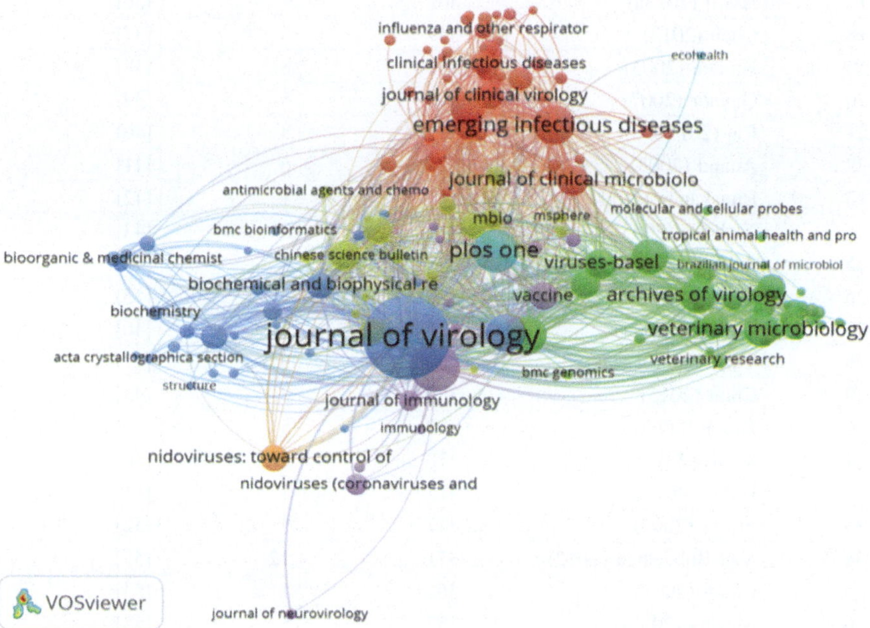

Fig. 5 Source and citations relationship of the sources that published documents on coronavirus research (N.B.: (1) Sources that have published at least ten documents were considered)

Table 5 Top documents that have been cited for at least 300 times

Id	Document	Citations	Links	References
1	Ksiazek (2003)	1891	23	[21]
2	Drosten (2003)	1802	18	[22]
3	Rota (2003)	1507	22	[23]
4	Peiris (2003a)	1472	18	[24]
5	Zaki (2012)	1353	13	[25]
6	Marra (2003)	1298	17	[26]
7	Allander (2005)	1037	5	[20]
8	Li (2003)	1009	11	[27]
9	Guan (2003)	918	10	[28]
10	Li (2005a)	877	9	[29]
11	Peiris (2003b)	852	7	[30]
12	Van Der Hoek (2004)	768	17	[31]
13	Snijder (2003)	686	15	[32]
14	Poutanen (2003)	678	9	[33]
15	Lau (2005)	658	15	[34]
16	Woo (2005)	658	15	[35]
17	Assiri (2013a)	562	7	[36]
18	Chen (2013)	549	2	[37]
19	Kuiken (2003)	499	8	[38]
20	Gaynor (2007)	496	5	[39]
21	Raj (2013)	492	8	[40]
22	Anand (2003)	473	6	[41]
23	Ruuskanen (2011)	461	1	[42]
24	Nicholls (2003)	412	3	[43]
25	Allander (2007)	397	4	[44]
26	Imai (2005)	390	5	[45]
27	Traggiai (2004)	389	4	[46]
28	Thiel (2003)	388	9	[47]
29	Chou (2015)	385	2	[48]
30	Bosch (2003)	380	5	[49]
31	Assiri (2013b)	378	2	[50]
32	Daffis (2010)	377	1	[51]
33	Fraser (2004)	377	2	[52]
34	Van Boheemen (2012)	371	12	[53]
35	Cinatl (2003)	362	1	[54]
36	Meyers (2005)	357	5	[55]
37	Reusken (2013)	353	3	[56]
38	Hota (2004)	349	0	[57]
39	Woo (2012)	338	10	[58]
40	Fouchier (2004)	338	16	[59]
41	Stevenson (2013)	336	1	[60]

(continued)

Table 5 (continued)

Id	Document	Citations	Links	References
42	Song (2012)	335	2	[61]
43	Yang (2003)	335	5	[62]
44	Chou (2003)	329	1	[63]
45	Zuest (2011)	323	2	[64]
46	Yang (2004)	322	6	[65]
47	Li (2005b)	313	7	[66]
48	Van Elden (2001)	309	0	[67]
49	Wang (2003)	308	4	[68]
50	Ge (2013)	306	6	[69]
51	Simmons (2005)	306	3	[70]
52	Azhar (2014)	305	4	[71]
53	Knoops (2008)	303	2	[72]

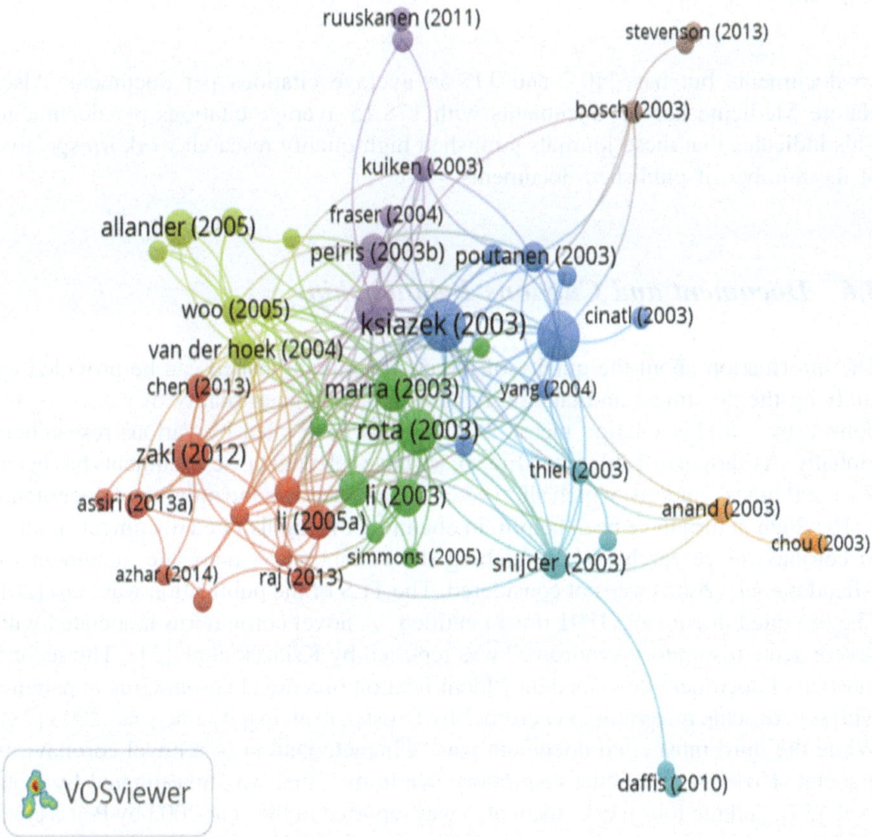

Fig. 6 Documents and citations relationship of the publications that have been cited for at least 300 times

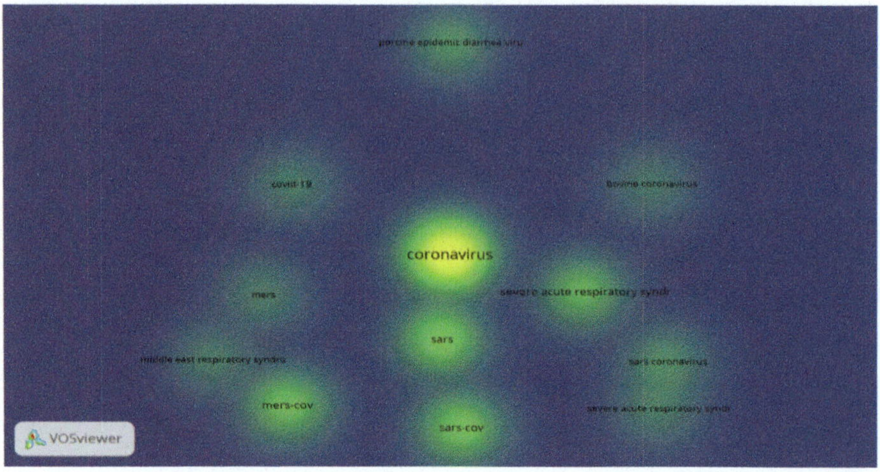

Fig. 7 Density visualization map of the coronavirus, major coronavirus-related infections and symptoms

16 documents but has 240.2 and 118.56 average citations per document. Also, Nature Medicine has 13 documents with 178.15 average citations per document. This indicates that these journals published high-quality research work irrespective of the number of published documents.

3.6 Document and Citations Relationship

The information about the quality of the documents published can be provided by studying the document and citation relationship. A higher quality of work is symbolized by a higher citation metric and thus has been cited by various researchers globally. As shown in Table 5 and Fig. 6, we have selected those documents having at least 300 times citations, which allowed us to narrow down the number of documents to 10 which in turn have been helpful in obtaining the highly cited documents related to coronavirus research. While fetching the collaboration map, the document by Allander et al. (2005) was not considered. The TLS of the publication was zero [20]. The top-cited document (1891 times) entitled "A novel coronavirus associated with severe acute respiratory syndrome" was reported by Ksiazek et al. [21]. The second most cited document described the "Identification of a novel coronavirus in patients with severe acute respiratory syndrome" by Drosten et al. in the same year, 2003 [22]. While the third most cited document was "Characterization of a novel coronavirus associated with severe acute respiratory syndrome" that was investigated by Rota et al. [23], and the fourth document also was reported in the year 2003 by Peiris et al. (2003) entitled "Coronavirus as a possible cause of the severe acute respiratory syndrome" [24]. Thereafter, the publication by Zaki Ali Moh [25] received a good number of citations. The topic of the study was "Isolation of a Novel coronavirus from a man with pneumonia in Saudi Arabia." This means that these are the five documents that are followed by other high-quality documents in the research area of coronavirus.

Funding Agencies

Any funding agency plays a very important role by supporting and promoting research and development work in any specific area. Funding is among the most important pillars who is responsible for the growth of any subject area. Thus, we have extracted in total the top twenty global funding agencies who have supported funding in the area of coronavirus research as depicted in table S4. The United States Department of Health and Human Services (HSS) acquires the first position with the contribution of 17.58% of total research among 1628 documents related to the coronavirus research. It was followed by the National Institutes of Health (NIH), USA, being in the second position with 17.10% from 1583 documents. National Council for Scientific and Technological Development (CNPq) is being in the 20th position with 69 documents and 0.745%.

3.7 Identifying Coronavirus Infections and Health Condition by Density Visualization Map

The density visualization map was created by co-occurrence and analysis of the keywords (Fig. 7). Screenings of the keywords were done manually, such that only coronavirus and associated clinical symptoms or disease terms are selected for the density visualization map generation. The density visualization map analysis suggested that the coronavirus-related diseases are associated with severe acute respiratory syndrome. This is suggestive of the fact that even though there is a mutation in the coronavirus, which changes its characteristics, all of them precipitate severe acute respiratory syndrome.

4 Conclusion

In light of the results of the scientometric analysis of the research paper, in the area of the coronavirus, there was a significant increase in various aspects, which includes the number of author appearances, number of multi-authored articles, etc. In gist, the information on 9257 number of documents related to the above-mentioned research area was extracted from the Web of Science. The extracted information was then used to perform a detailed scientometric analysis. It was observed that the research in this field of study started as early at 2000, but the research in the said field started receiving much attention post-2000. Since then from 2000 till 2020, research articles published reached a number of 9257. It was found that most of the economically developed countries were involved in the research related to the coronavirus. Also, the USA published the most number of documents followed by China. The USA had a TLS of 1941 indicating that the country was involved in extensive collaborative research. In terms of collaboration, China was in the second position. The University of Hong Kong was in the first position and was the most influential and impactful organization, having worked in the mentioned field of research with 417 documents with 56.62 average citations and TLS of 384, followed by Chinese Academy of Sciences with 306 documents, 33.80 citations, and 283 TLS. Other organizations like the Centers for Disease Control and Prevention, Utrecht University, Chinese Academy of Agricultural Sciences, The Chinese University of Hong Kong, and The University of North Carolina also received good attention from the researchers. The research groups of Yuen Kwok-Yung, followed by Ralph S. Baric and Christian Drosten, had the highest number of documents of 6176, 3843 and 5614, respectively. The scope for research collaboration across the globe is really very large, which, in turn, would definitely help in improving the overall research quality on coronavirus. The "Journal of Virology" has the highest number of 886 documents that have been published till date, and the documents were able to gain 39,407 citations for the journal. The journal "Virology" occupied the second spot by publishing 285 numbers of documents with 7759 citations. The top-cited document entitled "A novel coronavirus associated with severe acute respiratory syndrome" was reported by Ksiazek et al. (2003), which was found to be the most impactful documents in terms of average citations per documents. The document described as "Identification of a novel coronavirus in patients with severe acute respiratory syndrome" was cited as the second most by Drosten C et al. in the same year. United States Department of Health and Human Services is the highest supporter funding agency in coronavirus research among all other agencies globally.

Acknowledgements All the authors are thankful for their institutional support.

Competing Interests The authors report no conflicts of interest in this work.

Author Contributions All the authors contributed to data collection, drafting, editing, or revising the article gave final approval of the version to be published and agree to be accountable for all aspects of the work.

Referrences

1. Zhou F et al (2020) Clinical course and risk factors for mortality of adult inpatients with COVID-19 in Wuhan, China: a retrospective cohort study. The Lancet
2. Sohrabi C et al (2020) World health organization declares global emergency: a review of the 2019 novel coronavirus (COVID-19). Int J Surgery

3. Walls AC et al (2020) Structure, function, and antigenicity of the SARS-CoV-2 spike glycoprotein. Cell
4. Zhong N et al (2003) Epidemiology and cause of severe acute respiratory syndrome (SARS) in Guangdong. People's Republic of China. Lancet 362(9393):1353–1358
5. de Groot RJ et al (2013) Commentary: Middle East respiratory syndrome coronavirus (MERS-CoV): announcement of the Coronavirus Study Group. J Virology 87(14):7790–7792
6. Makino S, Joo M, Makino JK (1991) A system for study of coronavirus mRNA synthesis: a regulated, expressed subgenomic defective interfering RNA results from intergenicsite insertion. J Virology 65(11):6031–6041
7. Liu C et al (2020) Research and development on therapeutic agents and vaccines for COVID-19 and related human coronavirus diseases. ACS Central Science 6(3)315–331
8. Gallagher TM (1996) Murine coronavirus membrane fusion is blocked by modification of thiols buried within the spike protein. J Virology 70(7):4683–4690
9. Li F et al (2005) Structure of SARS coronavirus spike receptor-binding domain complexed with receptor. Sci 309(5742):1864–1868
10. Han Y, Yang H (2020) The transmission and diagnosis of 2019 novel coronavirus infection disease (COVID-19): a Chinese perspective. J Med Virology
11. Paules CI, Marston HD, Fauci AS (2020) Coronavirus infections—more than just the common cold. Jama 323(8):707–708
12. Nikhra V, Exploring pathophysiology of COVID-19 infection: faux espoir and dormant therapeutic options
13. Chen Z-M et al (2020) Diagnosis and treatment recommendations for pediatric respiratory infection caused by the 2019 novel coronavirus. World J Pediatrics 1–7
14. Zhang H et al (2020) Angiotensin-converting enzyme 2 (ACE2) as a SARS-CoV-2 receptor: molecular mechanisms and potential therapeutic target. Intensive Care Medicine 1–5
15. Li Z, Huang Y, Guo X (2020) The brain, another potential target organ, needs early protection from SARS-CoV-2 neuroinvasion. Sci China Life Sci 1
16. Ashour HM et al (2020) Insights into the recent 2019 novel Coronavirus (SARS-CoV-2) in light of past human coronavirus outbreaks. Pathogens 9(3):186
17. Xu Y-H, et al (2020) Clinical and computed tomographic imaging features of novel coronavirus pneumonia caused by SARS-CoV-2. J Inf
18. Yang Y et al (2019) Abibliometric review of laboratory safety in universities. Safety Sci 120:14–24
19. van Eck NJ, Waltman L (2010) Software survey: VOSviewer, a computer program for bibliometric mapping. Scientometric 84(2):523–538
20. Allander T et al (2005) Cloning of a human parvovirus by molecular screening of respiratory tract samples. Proceed Nat Academy Sci United States America 102(36):12891
21. Ksiazek TG et al (2003) A novel coronavirus associated with severe acute respiratory syndrome. New England J Med 348(20):1953–1966
22. Drosten C et al (2003) Identification of a novel coronavirus in patients with severe acute respiratory syndrome. New England J Med 348(20)1967–1976
23. Rota PA et al (2003) Characterization of a novel coronavirus associated with severe acute respiratory syndrome. Sci 300(5624):1394
24. Peiris JSM et al (2003) Coronavirus as a possible cause of severe acute respiratory syndrome. Lancet 361(9366):1319–1325
25. ZakiAM et al (2012) Isolation of a novel coronavirus from a man with pneumonia in Saudi Arabia. New England J Med 367(19):1814–1820
26. Marra MA et al (2003) The genome sequence of the SARS associated coronavirus. Sci 300 (5624):1399
27. Li W et al (2003) Angiotensin-converting enzyme 2 is a functional receptor for the SARS coronavirus. Nature 426(6965):450–454
28. Guan Y et al (2003) Isolation and characterization of viruses related to the SARS coronavirus from animals in Southern hina. Sci 302(5643):276
29. Li W et al (2005) Bats are natural reservoirs of SARS-like coronaviruses. Sci 310(5748):676

30. Peiris JSM et al (2003) Clinical progression and viral load in a community outbreak of coronavirus-associated SARS pneumonia: a prospective study. Lancet 361(9371):1767–1772
31. van der Hoek L et al (2004) Identification of a new human coronavirus. Nature Med 10(4):368–373
32. Snijder EJ et al (2003) Unique and conserved features of genome and proteome of SARS coronavirus, an early split-off from the coronavirus group 2 lineage. J Mole Biol 331(5):991–1004
33. Poutanen SM et al (2003) Identification of severe acute respiratory syndrome in Canada. New England J Med 348(20):1995–2005
34. Lau SKP et al (2005) Severe acute respiratory syndrome coronavirus-like virus in Chinese horseshoe bats. Proceed National Academy Sci United States Am 102(39):14040
35. Woo PCY et al (2005) Characterization and complete genome sequence of a novel coronavirus, coronavirus HKU1, from patients with pneumonia. J Virology 79(2):884
36. Assiri A et al (2013) Hospital outbreak of Middle East respiratory syndrome coronavirus. New England J Med 369(5):407–416
37. Chen Y et al (2013) Human infections with the emerging avian influenza A H7N9 virus from wet market poultry: clinical analysis and characterisation of viral genome. Lancet 381 (9881):1916–1925
38. Kuiken T et al (2003) Newly discovered coronavirus as the primary cause of severe acute respiratory syndrome. Lancet 362(9380):263–270
39. GaynorAM et al (2007) Identification of a novel polyomavirus from patients with acute respiratory tract infections. PLoS Pathogens 3(5)
40. Raj VS et al (2013) Dipeptidyl peptidase 4 is a functional receptor for the emerging human coronavirus-EMC. Nature 495(7440):251–254
41. Anand K et al (2003) Coronavirus main proteinase ($3CL^{pro}$) structure: basis for design of anti-SARS drugs. Sci 300(5626):1763
42. Ruuskanen O et al (2011) Viral pneumonia. Lancet 377(9773):1264–1275
43. Nicholls JM et al (2003) Lung pathology of fatal severe acute respiratory syndrome. Lancet 361(9371):1773–1778
44. Allander T et al (2007) Human bocavirus and acute wheezing in children. Clinical Infect Diseases 44(7):904–910
45. Imai Y et al (2005) Angiotensin-converting enzyme 2 protects from severe acute lung failure. Nature 436(7047):112–116
46. Traggiai E et al (2004) An efficient method to make human monoclonal antibodies from memory B cells: potent neutralization of SARS coronavirus. Nature Med 10(8):871–875
47. Thiel V et al (2003) Mechanisms and enzymes involved in SARS coronavirus genome expression. J General Virology 84(9):2305–2315
48. Kuo-Chen C (2015) Impacts of bioinformatics to medicinal chemistry. Med Chem 11(3):218–234
49. Bosch BJ et al (2003) The coronavirus spike protein Is a class I virus fusion protein: structural and functional characterization of the fusion core complex. J Virology 77(16):8801
50. Assiri A et al (2013) Epidemiological, demographic, and clinical characteristics of 47 cases of Middle East respiratory syndrome coronavirus disease from Saudi Arabia: a descriptive study. Lancet Infect Diseases 13(9):752–761
51. Daffis S et al (2010) 2'-O methylation of the viral mRNA capevades host restriction by IFIT family members. Nature 468(7322):452–456
52. Fraser C et al (2004) Factors that make an infectious disease outbreak controllable. Proceed Nat Academy Sci United States Am 101(16):6146
53. van Boheemen S et al (2012) Genomic characterization of a newly discovered coronavirus associated with acute respiratory distress syndrome in Humans. mBio 3(6):e00473–12
54. Cinatl J et al (2003) Glycyrrhizin, an active component of liquorice roots, and replication ofSARS-associated coronavirus. Lancet 361(9374):2045–2046
55. Meyers LA et al (2005) Network theory and SARS: predicting outbreak diversity. J Theoret Biol 232(1):71–81

56. Reusken CBEM et al (2013) Middle East respiratory syndrome coronavirus neutralising serum antibodies in dromedary camels: a comparative serological study. Lancet Infect Diseases 13(10):859–866
57. Weinstein RA, Hota B (2004) Contamination, disinfection, and cross-colonization: are hospital surfacesreservoirs for nosocomial infection? Clinical Infect Diseases 39(8):1182–1189
58. Woo PCY et al, Discovery of seven novel mammalian and avian coronaviruses in the genus deltacoronavirus supports bat coronaviruses as the gene source of alpha coronavirus and beta coronavirus and avian coronaviruses as the gene source of gamma coronavirus and deltacoronavirus

The manufacturer's authorised representative in the EU is Springer Nature Customer Service Centre GmbH, Europaplatz 3, 69115 Heidelberg, Germany. If you have any concerns regarding our products, please contact ProductSafety@springernature.com

Printed and bound by CPI Group (UK) Ltd, Croydon, CR0 4YY
30/09/2026
02225293-0001